The Prostate

Everything You Need to Know About the Man Gland

Cover design: Debbie Geltner

Cover image: Getty Images: Hercules and Cacus (detail), Baccio Bandinelli.

Book design and typesetting: WildElement.ca

Author photo: Toru Kawasaki

Library and Archives Canada Cataloguing in Publication

Taguchi, Yosh, author

The prostate : everything you need to know about the man gland / by Dr. Yosh Taguchi. -- Revised edition.

Revision of: The prostate : everything you need to know about the man gland / Yosh Taguchi ; introduction by Adrian Waller. -- Toronto : Key Porter, c2001.

Issued in print and electronic formats.

ISBN 978-1-927535-35-6 (pbk.).-- ISBN 978-1-927535-36-3 (html).--
ISBN 978-1-927535-37-0 (html).--ISBN 978-1-927535-38-7 (pdf)
    1. Prostate--Diseases--Popular works. I. Title.
RC899.T33 2014   616.6'5   C2013-907835-5
                                       C2013-907836-3

Printed and bound in Canada by Marquis Book Printing.

Legal Deposit, National Library and Archives Canada
et Dépôt légal, Bibliothèque et archives nationales du Québec.

Linda Leith Publishing acknowledges the support of the
Canada Council for the Arts and of SODEC.

Linda Leith Publishing
P.O. Box 322, Station Victoria
Westmount, Quebec H3Z 2V8 Canada
www.lindaleith.com

The Prostate

Everything You Need to Know About the Man Gland

REVISED EDITION

DR. YOSH TAGUCHI

To my family

CONTENTS

1

Foreword

The overriding emotion is terror. The surgeon is kind. He is considerate. He is painfully aware of your distress. At the same time, the diagnosis of prostate cancer is a blow to the gut, light-years away from the diagnosis of benign prostatic hyperplasia, or simple enlargement, which you had so desperately hoped for.

"What will happen to me? What can I do? Will I die? Will I become impotent? What is the five-year survival rate? What do I tell my wife? My kids? Why me?" These are only a few of the questions that come to mind at this terrible moment.

Yosh Taguchi is no stranger to this scenario, nor to all of these fearful questions. For more than fifty years, he has skillfully and patiently responded, reassured, treated, and often cured the tens of thousands of men who have sought his help with their prostate problems. He has removed diseased prostates, reduced the size of enlarged ones, and rebuilt structures, where necessary. A respected teacher and a surgical innovator, he has developed new and more effective procedures in the operating room, the Taguchi Loop being one in particular. Most importantly, however, he has also been a stalwart emotional support to every man he sees.

A quiet, self-effacing man, he seeks no public praise, and in fact, was almost at a loss for words when McGill University named a Chair in Urology in his honour only two years ago; a gift from a grateful and cured patient.

It's a long way from the crowded and difficult quarters of an internment camp for Japanese-Canadians to the offices, examining rooms and operating rooms of one of Canada's foremost surgical urologists. Yosh Taguchi has made this journey with dignity and aplomb. It is not so much what he does, but who he is that distinguishes this physician from the pack. There are few doctors whose patients would be willing to wait for hours to see them, without complaint, but Dr. Taguchi's waiting room is filled with patient men who know that the good doctor will take all the time he needs with them.

Yosh Taguchi treats the whole man and not just the symptoms. He is intimately acquainted with his patients' histories, their families, their expectations, and their fears, and he addresses all of them with each visit. From an unassuming set of examining rooms and an office on the sixth floor of Montreal's Royal Victoria Hospital, he hands out advice, prescriptions, humour, and hope, all the while performing gold-standard examinations and procedures.

Each man in his office feels that he is the only patient that morning. Each man firmly believes that this doctor, *his* doctor, will find the most effective way to treat his condition, and each man also knows for sure that, at some time after the examination, Yosh Taguchi will point to a huge stack of books sitting on the corner of his desk and casually ask "Have you read my latest one yet?"

Yosh is my urologist, my golfing partner, my model for humility, and my good friend. He is a power in the medical field, but my greatest tribute to him is that he is, simply, a good man. This book represents a lifetime of his work and study. It's a must read for every man who has, or used to have a prostate.

Howard M. Schwartz, B.A. M.Ed.
Editor

Howard M. Schwartz is a retired educational administrator who now consults in strategic planning and organizational success for school boards, administrators, and industries. He is also a professional speechwriter.

Author's Note

The first edition of *The Prostate*, which was published in 2001, was the brainchild of Anna Porter, publisher of Key Porter Books. She thought there should be a popular book on the prostate and that I should be the one to write it. She might have been influenced by the fact that I had written a book on seldom-mentioned medical problems called *Private Parts*, which became an international best seller.

The Prostate was well received in Canadian, American, and British editions. It was also translated into French, *La Prostate* published by Guérin Éditeur, and Spanish, *La Prostata* published by Amat.

Twelve years have passed and, sadly, Key Porter Books no longer exists. I felt there was enough material for a second edition, and when I approached Linda Leith she was enthusiastic and highly supportive of the project.

The Canadian author Adrian Waller helped me with the first edition. I spent many weekends at his home working on the book with Adrian, while his wife, Irene, served us snacks and tea. Adrian has since retired to Ontario. Howard Schwartz, who was my editor for *Zen in Action*, my third book, agreed to be my editor for this revised edition of *The Prostate*. His input has been invaluable, bringing life to often lifeless pages.

In recent years a number of Canadian and American experts have authored books on the prostate. I have examined them, found them current and comprehensive, but a chore to read. I hope my good friend Fred Lowy is right when he says mine is a page turner.

Yosh Taguchi, MD, PhD, FRCSC
Montreal

1

The Nature of the Beast

Of all the glands in the male body, none can be more aggravating than a small, inconspicuous mass that surrounds the urethra as it exits the bladder. This seemingly harmless collection of glandular cells, muscle tissue, and supporting structures has been at the core of male middle-aged angst from the beginnings of medicine as we know it.

This book will devote itself to the description, analysis, treatment and even the removal of the "man gland" – the prostate. Sometimes praised, often maligned, universally feared, this tiny structure will dictate the course of old age in many, if not most men, worldwide.

Not long ago, one of the hundred or so patients I see each week at Montreal's Royal Victoria Hospital, where I have been practising Urology for close to half a century, asked me, "Why do I have a prostate, doc?"

I was a little taken aback by his question. No one had ever asked it of me before. "I mean," the patient went on, "I know why I've got an elbow, a thyroid, and a penis, and I know they're all useful. But no doctor has yet been able to tell me why I have a prostate. Oh, they can all tell me the problems I'm having with my prostate, but I'm still waiting for one of them to explain why I have this gland in the first place. What does it do? What is it there for? Can I live without it?"

I thought for a moment before telling the patient exactly what I have been telling my students at McGill University, where I have been lecturing on urology for the same length of time: that this small, walnut-sized gland that sits at the neck of the bladder where it meets the urethra, behind the pubic bone and in front of the rectum, weighing a mere 20 grams when it is healthy, has a very limited use which, as we will see, diminishes with a man's age.

It is needed most when a man is in his younger years and wants to impregnate a woman, or when he is merely seeking to exercise his sexual prowess. Nonetheless, the prostate gland is not a "prostitute" gland, as another of my patients used to call it. Nor is it the "prostrate," which is how less-aware men and women tended to term it before the gland found itself at the centre of so many news reports that focus on it today.

To remember the difference, I used to tell my students, "The man lay prostrate in his bed waiting for the doctor to examine his prostate." They quickly saw the difference and laughed. Prostate problems, however, are no laughing matter, as those students well knew.

NORMAL MALE ANATOMY

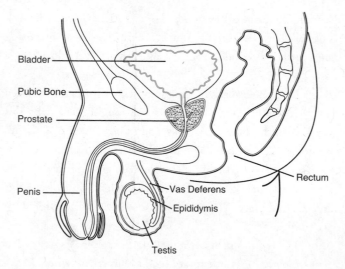

6

It isn't always that way, of course. In a young boy, the gland is vestigial or undetectable – almost non-existent – lying like a cluster of seeds under the lining of the urinary tract. Most boys, I venture to say, don't even know they have the beginnings of a prostate gland that may grow to haunt them later.

At puberty, though, this anatomy begins to change. The surge of the male hormone, testosterone, which heralds manhood, stimulates these seeds to germinate and grow. The boy's external sex organs – the penis, the testicles, and the scrotum – also enlarge under the influence of the male hormone as he becomes a man. Now he has a prostate gland.

FORMATION OF THE PROSTATE

In essence, the development of this gland resembles the growth of a softwood tree with its many branches. In fact, because of this similarity, the growing process has been called "arborization," a term borrowed from botanists. Twenty such trees may be involved in this process, but a closer look at the end product suggests the growth to be closer in appearance to that of a patch of raspberry bushes.

The berries represent the little glandular structures within the larger prostate (called acini by the pathologists), and the stem and leaves make up the supporting tissue, called stroma, which is fibromuscular. In a normal prostate, the glandular component makes up twenty percent, and the muscle cells forty percent of the total mass. The balance, or the last forty percent, consists of tissue fluid.

Remember the raspberry bush analogy because I will come back to it later when I discuss prostate enlargement and, of course, the much more serious ailment, prostate cancer – the nightmare or dread of every man alive.

PROSTATE GLAND STRUCTURE

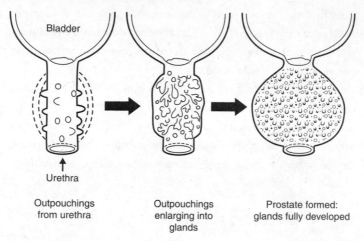

Bladder

Urethra

Outpouchings
from urethra

Outpouchings
enlarging into
glands

Prostate formed:
glands fully developed

Thankfully, most men never get this awful disease, but statistical evidence does not prevent them from feeling anxiety about what may happen to their prostate glands as they age. In fact, it is true to say that almost all males over forty worry now and then about this part of their anatomy, and while a lot of this worry is disease related, a good part of it may be purely psychological.

The prostate gland produces a protein called prostate specific antigen, or PSA. When sperm from the testicles and fluid from the seminal vesicles are sent into the prostate, it joins up with the prostatic secretion and a protein specific to it called the PSA, to make what we know as the gelatinous ejaculate. Later, the PSA transforms that sticky substance into a distinctly liquid form, which is important in the fertilization process.

Actually, the prostate secretes sixty percent of the ejaculate. Or, to put it another way, it makes the bulk of the fluid in which the spermatozoa – or the sperm that is ejaculated on orgasm – is contained.

This prostatic fluid, however, is not essential for sperm maturation or for sperm survival. In fact, the sperm extracted from the epididymis, where it exits from the testicle, can create a normal pregnancy on its own, without needing to pass through the prostate. So, neither the PSA nor the seminal vesicles found behind the gland actually need to figure in the fertilization process. We know, for example, that we can draw sperm directly from the testicle or epididymis by syringe for impregnation, long before it even reaches the prostate. This, in fact, is what is done in assisted reproduction.

Nonetheless, it is vital for the sperm to be in this medium when natural impregnation is the goal. Ironically, then, when a man reaches middle-age and no longer wants to impregnate a woman, he really has no further use for this gland at all, yet it can cause him more mental anguish, more emotional aggravation, indeed, more bitterness and anger, than any other part of his body.

Accordingly, millions of men the world over ask their urologists the same questions:

- Will my prostate grow and choke my urine flow?
- Will it become cancerous?
- Will surgery or radiotherapy become necessary and leave me wetting my pants or unable to get an erection, or both?
- Will the diagnosis of cancer be missed and lead me to live my life in excruciating pain?
- Will the cancer spread into my bones?
- Will the doctors bungle the job of curing me, no matter what the problem?
- Will my prostate eventually kill me, as my uncle's killed him?
- How can I protect myself from the severest prostate problems?

The main cause of many of the problems that afflict the gland is in its design, which is flawed indeed. Ideally, the prostate should have been given an external drainage pipe – such as one fitted to a testicle or a salivary gland – that would help any unwanted inflammation or in-

9

fection drain away naturally, but it doesn't have anything like this at all.

If it were a globular gland with an external drainage system, its enlargement, which we will discuss in detail later, would not choke the urinary passage and could be left alone, and any cancerous growth could simply be snipped out easily without the need for major reconstructive surgery. Instead, the prostate gland is wrapped *around* the urethra, with an *internal* drainage pipe that is joined by the sperm duct close to its opening, and this means that rather delicate surgery may be required to repair a severely diseased prostate.

As some men who have had their prostate glands removed can testify, it is truly an organ they can live without. This means that, providing there are no other urinary problems involved, a man who doesn't have a prostate can still enjoy life to its fullest, with relatively few side effects. This may come as a surprise to many people but, like a lot of the men on whom I have performed this radical operation, I can vouch that it is true.

I routinely ask all of my patients who have had their cancerous prostates removed, "Surely there must be some subtle way your life is different now compared to what it was before the surgery?"

Usually, this puzzles them, and they reply, "No, doc. There's really no difference."

Indeed, without a prostate gland, urination can be just as normal, a sex life just as satisfactory, and orgasm just as intense. Much less fluid, however, is ejaculated, which is what I meant when I said that most middle-aged men did not really need the prostate to function as nature had originally intended. In this way, the prostate can be a tenacious little beast, and, when enlarged or inflamed, the source of a disproportionate amount of distress.

Finally, please remember PSA. The increased production of this protein is used as a marker both for the diagnosis of cancer and the possible reoccurrence of it after treatment. You will find that as this book progresses, I will refer to it often.

2

Examining the Prostate

The term prostate comes from the Greek *prostates*, which means "one that stands before." Did the Greeks think that the prostate "stood" before the bladder? Or did they mean that it preceded the penis? Whatever was intended, it seems that the ancient Greeks were almost as uncertain about this enigmatic and inaccessible gland as we are today.

If you go to a doctor with a sore finger, toe, or elbow, he or she can see it, touch it, even squeeze it if necessary. That is to say, the physician can examine it in such a fashion as to be fairly certain what is wrong with it and what should be done to treat it. The prostate, however, is a different matter because it is so deeply set within the pelvic area and because it often requires more than one diagnostic procedure to ascertain what ails it.

Consider the three blind men who were asked to describe an elephant. The first felt the tusk and described the animal as being rock hard. The second stroked the animal's leg and thought it was tough and rough. The third felt its ears and thought the animal was soft and velvety. The story serves to tell us that if we rely on only one method of examining something, we can make similar errors in judgment.

There are a number of ways we urologists examine the prostate:

- The digital rectal examination;
- The cystoscopy;

- Various imaging techniques, such as the trans-rectal ultra-sound examination, the CT scan, or the multiparametric magnetic resonance imaging (MRI); and
- A blood test called the PSA.

We are also guided by what the patient tells us about his family history, his occupation, and medical problems – and what he may say in any one of several standardized questionnaires that are used to elicit more specific diagnostic information. These forms invariably ask about the quality and regularity of the patient's urination, if his urine is discoloured or foul-smelling, which may denote an infection, how many times he urinates in the night, how easy it is for him to start the flow or stop it, if he sees blood at the beginning or at the end or thoughout urination, and if he is able to have an erection.

We may also use techniques to measure a patient's actual urine flow and bladder function – tests called urodynamic studies. These, however, usually come after the more standard investigative procedures.

When cancer is detected, even more examining techniques are used, and I will discuss these in their appropriate places. Meanwhile, I will concentrate on the basic tests that should be done either as a matter of routine or that are administered for diagnosis when a patient complains that he is not urinating properly or is feeling pain in the prostatic region.

THE DIGITAL RECTAL EXAMINATION

In this procedure, both swift and relatively pain-free, the doctor places his or her gloved and lubricated index finger into the rectum and feels the back surface of the prostate through the front wall of the rectum.

The Canadian guidelines for family doctors do not consider this test mandatory. General Norman Schwarzkopf, commander of Operation Desert Storm, must have been forever grateful that his physician, an American military medical officer, had not been subjected to any such rule, because it was the digital rectal examination that detected his early prostate cancer. His PSA reading at the time was 2.1. The General's life—he died of pneumonia in December 2012—testifies to the fact that blood tests alone are often not enough to detect prostate problems; the earliest signs of these are often detected with the rectal examination, which all men aged over forty should have at regular intervals, the frequency depending upon the initial assessment.

Doctors who do the test usually have the patient lie on his side curled up in the foetal position, or ask him to assume a position wherein his elbows, chest, and knees are on the examining table. I, and many other urologists, prefer to do the rectal exam with the patient standing, feet apart, bent forward, with his elbows on the table. It is, perhaps, a crude position, but I find that it provides the fullest possible access to the gland.

Once the patient is in position, I place my lubricated index finger flat against the anus, and this causes the sphincter to relax. When I feel this relaxation, I glide the finger in carefully.

When the patient is in the standing position, my finger can probe more deeply, and I can quickly tell if the right side of his gland feels exactly the same as the left, as it should. Of course, the most important point in doing the rectal examination is to search for any unusual firm, even rock hard, surfaces that would suggest the patient might have a tumour. Briefly, while examining a patient when he is standing, I can complete the procedure in a matter of seconds, and he is usually happy about that.

I have yet to find a patient who enjoys this examination. Some patients joke about it, saying, "Does your mother know what you do for a living?"

A good-natured middle-aged patient, who was also known to be a joker, commented after his rectal examination, "Well, doc, you have convinced me of one thing."

"What's that?" I asked, somewhat naively.

"You've convinced me to stay with my wife."

I am often asked how I could possibly remember the size of a patient's prostate from one year to the next, when I must be doing thousands of examinations every year. My notes indicate my guess of the size of the gland, and whether it was soft, rubbery, firm, irregular, or if it contained other indicators that something might be wrong.

Also, many patients ask me how I can detect a tumour that might be on the other side of the gland, when my examining finger can feel only the back surface. My response is quite simple. Seventy percent of all cancers originate in the area of the prostate that is easily accessible to me.

CYSTOSCOPY

It's true to say, I think, that every man dreads the thought of an instrument the thickness of a pencil being inserted into his penis all the way into his bladder. Some men are so fearful of another cystoscopy that they have been known to abandon follow-up care. Other patients have written about their ordeals.

I recall one disquieting, yet entertaining article on this subject that appeared some years ago in *Esquire* magazine. Cystoscopy and vasectomy qualify as popular topics for masochistic confessions, but not always for good reason.

One of my patients, who has a bladder problem, has had innumerable cystoscopic examinations. He tells me, "I don't mind the procedure at all because I know that it gets to the heart of the problem. If the urologist is as gentle as you are, it doesn't hurt much at all. It's a little uncomfortable when you move that thing around, but other than that it's not hard to take." Actually, some urologists are considerably gentler than others. I'd stay away from a urologist who says, "It's gonna hurt, so let's get it over with quickly."

A gentle urologist will lubricate the passage into the penis with a generous glob of lubricant that contains a mild local anaesthetic called xylocaine. He or she will then insert the cystoscope slowly. As the instrument passes through the sphincter, which keeps the urine in the bladder, a little bit of discomfort is usually inevitable, though short-lived.

A nervous patient who cannot relax his muscles is likely to feel more pain. Sensation is also felt as the instrument passes through the prostatic urethra – that is, the urinary passage through the prostate itself. There is only mild discomfort once the instrument is in the bladder.

Without removing the shaft from the patient's urethra, the urologist can insert lenses that allow him to inspect the bladder from various angles. A zero lens enables the doctor to look straight ahead, a thirty-degree lens allows him to look down thirty degrees, and with a seventy-degree lens, he can examine at an angle of seventy degrees. By changing the lens, the urologist can inspect both the urinary passage and the bladder quite thoroughly.

The introduction of a flexible cystoscope means that the cystoscopy can be carried out without positioning the patient as for childbirth – that is to say, with his legs draped over stirrups. Finger controls allow the urologist to snake the instrument in the direction he or she desires, and, as the instrument is smaller in calibre, it is less distressing to the patient. The field of vision the flexible cystoscope provides is narrower, however, and this means that the examination might not be as thorough. Sometimes, the traditional instrument, which is a lot older than most practising urologists, can be a more exacting method.

A cystoscopy used to be a routine examination for prostate assessment. Today, we administer cystoscope examinations only to those patients whose prostate troubles are accompanied by blood in the urine. Cystoscopy may detect either a bladder tumour or bladder stones. By this method, we can examine the prostatic ure-thra to ascertain if there is any obstruction, or "kissing" lobes, for a distance of up to five or six centimetres.

PROSTATE IMAGING

The prostate gland can be imaged indirectly, but somewhat incompletely, by a method called an intravenous pyelogram. In this test, the patient, who has been prepared by a bowel cleanout (enema), and dehydration (nothing to eat or drink after midnight), is injected intravenously with a contrast material that contains iodine. The fluid shows up on an X-ray as if it were bone. The dye is excreted by the kidney and outlines these as well as the ureters and bladder.

The final X-ray is taken after the patient has emptied his bladder. The urine retained in the bladder is called residual urine and the X-ray image will show this and any indentation on the floor of the bladder that may be caused by an enlarged prostate gland.

A computerized scan (CT scan) depicts the body as if it had been guillotined at different levels, half a centimetre apart. The test can be done with or without the injection of iodine. The cross-section image created by the computer reveals any lumps or bumps. The size and contour of the prostate can be seen during this procedure, but none of the finer details that we would see with either a magnetic scan or ultrasound.

The magnetic resonance scan provides much the same type of imaging, with more detail, and can suggest the presence or absence of cancer in the prostate. It is establishing itself as a test to do after the PSA or rectal examination suggests the possibility of cancer — before the ultrasound and ultrasound-guided biopsies.

Ultrasound imaging of the prostate gland, using a cigar-shaped probe that is inserted into the rectum, was introduced by Dr. Hiroki Watanabe of Kyoto, Japan. His original equipment was crude, indeed. The rotating probe was fixed to a chair and the patient was expected to actually impale himself upon it. The resulting image showed no more than bumps and lumps on the prostate's surface, but was unable to detect any other irregularities within the gland itself.

Dr. Watanabe's early audiences laughed and said, "Well, maybe this will work in the East," implying that Asian patients there were more stoic. His doubting colleagues did not realize that this was the beginning of a revolutionary advance in the assessment and examination of prostate problems – on a television screen.

The Japanese doctor's original equipment was crude in other ways. His probe used far fewer sound waves than those emitted by today's machines. The optimum vibration level of the sound waves for "seeing" the prostate is seven million vibrations per second. Interestingly, the human ear hears sound waves between twenty cycles and twenty-thousand cycles per second, while dogs can hear sounds of infinitely more than twenty-thousand cycles per second. The ultrasound waves "see" deep inside the gland as sound waves bounce off fat, glandular tissue, muscle, and cancerous tissue differently, and the results can be made to form telling images on the screen. This is because the bounce of sound waves off fat is quite different from their bounce off such solid tissue as the prostate gland itself.

By this method, the prostate can be measured in length, width, and height, and by multiplying the three measurements by a factor of 0.52 (a mathematical factor designed for a prostate-like shape), a volume measurement of the gland can be obtained. This would be most useful in determining what kind of surgery a patient may need – by incision or through the penis, with or without laser energy.

The gland itself is revealed on the television screen as a mottled grey organ, with the inner part clearly distinguishable from the outer part. Within the outer part there may be areas that look darker (hypoechoeic), or lighter (hyperechoeic). Again, this is of paramount use in detecting cancer, which is most often displayed as dark spots.

THE PSA

Finally, we come to the blood test known as the PSA – Prostate Specific Antigen – that protein I have told you about. This is secreted by every glandular prostate cell, and its function is to turn the gelatinous ejaculate matter into liquid. This simple blood test, which takes only a matter of seconds and requires no dieting or special preparation, has become a marker for prostate cancer. This is because most prostate cancer cells release ten times more PSA than non-cancerous prostate cells.

Confusing the issue are two facts: PSA counts will be higher when there is prostate enlargement, or prostate infection, and some cancers do not secrete the protein at all. Also, an elevated PSA does not necessarily denote the presence of cancer.

The perfect prostate cancer marker would be a measurable chemical that is released only by cancer cells on their own, and not by normal ones – so that when they are present there is a cancer, but when they are absent, there isn't. Alas, we have no such marker available – yet.

Every year new markers are proposed, but none of them has become fully established with the possible exception of PCA, a marker tested in a urine sample after prostate massage. This marker, along with the MRI, the magnetic scan, is changing how prostate cancer is diagnosed.

Such are the ways to diagnose prostate problems, and, as the years roll on, there will doubtless be more. As society ages and our clinics and hospitals are called upon to treat more and more urinary dysfunctions, new ways to see or feel the geography of this troublesome little gland will be in even greater demand.

3

ENLARGED PROSTATE:
The Signs and the Symptoms

Each year, urology clinics in virtually every major centre throughout Canada, the U.S., and around the world are jam-packed with men who complain they cannot urinate properly. Usually, this is because they have what urologists call benign prostatic hyperplasia. Simply put, this is a condition in which the prostate gland enlarges or swells and chokes the urethra.

The cause of this annoying problem can be manifold. Very often, it is simply because men have been taking off-the-shelf medications for coughs and colds. They might have taken Sudafed, Robidrine, Benylin, or Dristan, for example, or Sinutab, Novahistex, Robitussin, Actifed, or any other decongestant. Almost always they have neglected to read, or have ignored, the warnings on the package labels – that these medications should not be taken in the presence of symptoms of an enlarged prostate or any other urinary problem.

Understandably, then, some of my most grateful patients have been those for whom I have done nothing more than to provide temporary relief from an enlarged prostate, with the relatively simple passage of a catheter in their urethras – and a warning against all future use of decongestants.

It's worth mentioning here that one of the urologist's most valuable tools is a Foley catheter, so named because it was invented by an American doctor named Frederick E. B. Foley and first marketed as far back as 1934. Essentially, this is a two-channel length of flexible, hollow rubber tubing that allows urine, blood, and irrigating fluid to continuously drain from the bladder.

One channel in the wall of the catheter connects to a small balloon which, when inflated inside the bladder with 10 ml of water, prevents this ingenious draining system from falling out.

The catheter – it comes with a urine bag that is strapped to the leg, and which must be emptied from time to time – is used to temporarily drain the bladder in cases where normal urination is impossible, or more permanently for those patients who have lost control of their normal bladder functions. Many men must wear a Foley catheter while having treatment for severely enlarged prostates and prostatitis, sometimes before prostate surgery, and always after it.

Should the catheter plug with tissue or a blood clot, as is often the case in the early hours following surgery, manual irrigation is necessary. A little sterile water is pumped into the channel that drains the urine, and this is usually enough to ease the blockage. I have said that the Foley catheter is a rubber tubing, which is not totally correct. The rubber-like tube is often coated with silicone or made of silastic, a combination of rubber and silicone to which the body does not react. The catheter can come in varying calibres, have a third channel for continuous inflow of irrigating fluid, or have a hockey stick-like tip that makes its insertion easier in men with an enlarged prostate gland.

WHAT IS AN ENLARGED PROSTATE, AND HOW DOES IT GET THAT WAY?

The prostate gland is, as we have seen, a tiny structure that sprouts with the surge of the male hormone testosterone to become the size of a walnut in the adult male. The prostate is a gland that exists only to secrete fluid.

To understand how and why it enlarges, however, we must consider its composition again: One half of it consists of glandular cells, the other of a supporting framework that is composed largely of muscle cells and connective tissue. Imagine the prostate gland as a box of picked raspberries lying in a bed of straw. The berries are the glands, and the muscle cells the straw. In an enlarged prostate, there can be more or fewer berries as well as larger berries and/or more or less straw.

Generally speaking, when the enlargement is mostly glandular, or berry-like, the gland can grow to an enormous size without totally blocking the urinary stream. Overgrowth of the muscle cells, however, is likely to cause obstructive symptoms earlier. Of course, in many instances, the growth – or enlargement – is in both elements, which means that the urine flow is nearly always impaired.

It is easy to imagine how an enlarged prostate wrapped around the urinary passage can impede or block the flow of urine. The effect is similar to a kitchen sink that is slow to drain because debris is clinging to the walls of the pipe underneath it. In the same way, the urine spills slowly from the bladder when the passage is choked. Sometimes it is released in spurts, with stops along the way. Other times, the urine stream can be thin and require a lot of forcing.

But why does an enlarged prostate cause patients to void so often, with such urgency, and with such a frequent need as to interrupt sleep?

These irritative symptoms make sense if there is an associated urine infection, if there are stones in the bladder, or if the bladder does not empty out completely. Often, though, there are no such findings. All that is apparent is an enlarged gland and a frequent and urgent need to pass perfectly clear urine, particularly during the night.

Is it because the neck of the bladder is being stretched by the prostate and this stretching triggers the need to urinate? This seems like a logical explanation, but these same symptoms occur in older women,

21

and they have no prostate glands at all. Thus it is more likely the symptoms are from bladder irritation than from prostatic enlargement.

The bigger question is this: Why do so many prostate glands enlarge in middle age? The simple answer is that we don't really know. What we *do* know is that eunuchs, or males who underwent prepubertal castration, did not suffer from enlarged prostates. In other words, all those male sopranos who were castrated as boys in the Middle Ages were spared visits to urologists! All this is because castration eliminates what we call Leydid cells inside the testicles, and since these cells produce the testosterone, there has to be a causal link between an enlarged prostate and the presence of male hormones.

It is also true that this problem is more common in some parts of the world than in others, quite obviously implicating environmental factors and probably different diets and lifestyles. We also know that when men emigrate from areas where an enlarged prostate is uncommon – like Japan – to areas where it is very common, like the U.S., this geographical "protection" is lost within about twenty years.

The culprits are probably animal fats, and the protective foods are thought to be soy products. Fats are also thought to encourage prostate cancer, while soy beans are said to discourage it. Yet despite popular thinking among both patients and their wives, there appears to be no statistical link whatsoever between an enlarged prostate and prostate cancer. In other words, just because a man has an enlarged prostate does not by any stretch of the imagination mean that his gland is more likely to become cancerous.

To try to make this point – and prove that environment can be directly responsible for many causes of enlarged prostates – I have long lobbied for a study on those Caucasian men who have lived for more than twenty years in Japan. In this, I would hope to establish if – like their native Japanese friends who live alongside them in the same cities and with access to the same food – they too were relatively immune, not only from an enlarged prostate, but from prostate cancer, too. A decade has gone by, and I have not yet been able to get this study done.

What we know more definitely is that, statistically, enlarged prostate problems are also more common in certain families. Indeed, when they appear in men in their fifties, their brothers are four times more likely to require treatment for them, too. The reasons may be obvious: family members tend to share the same diet and the same lifestyles, not to mention similar genes, which may be genetically responsible for the problem.

At present, the genetic basis for an enlarged prostate is still being investigated, and the results are not yet known to us. More certain within the medical fraternity is that cells in an enlarged prostate contain more growth factors and appear to live longer, thus giving rise to the possibility that an enlarged prostate may be passed from father to son.

If a genetic explanation for this common ailment is likely, the specific gene, or genes, have yet to be identified. If and when they are, genetic engineering may well provide a cure for an enlarged prostate.

There was a time, about thirty years ago, when urologists deliberated very little before deciding how to treat a patient with an enlarged prostate. Nothing much was available to them. A patient who was complaining enough was encouraged to have the enlarged tissue carved out. So certain were urologists that the disease was progressive – that it would worsen and cause total urinary blockage – that even those patients who did not complain much were also advised to submit to surgery.

Indeed, only in the last three decades has it become apparent that an enlarged prostate was not necessarily progressive, and that its symptoms did not match prostate size – that a man could have a prostate like a grapefruit and have no blockage at all, yet another with a tangerine-sized gland might be unable to urinate at all, or be "in retention."

The term prostatism, which once meant symptoms from an enlarged prostate, is now being displaced by the term LUTS, which is short for Lower Urinary Tract Symptoms. Though the designation of a new term added little new insight, other things did.

FLOW STUDIES

Necessity has since become the mother of invention. What has emerged to date to add insight into the correlation between prostate size and urine flow are flow studies and ultrasound methods of measuring urinary retention.

In a flow study, the patient voids into a special funnel instead of into a urinal, and the amount of urine passed per unit time is recorded on a graph. In a normal male, the peak flow rate should exceed 15 ml per second. When the peak flow rate is under 10 ml per second, it suggests prostatic obstruction although a weakened bladder muscle or, in some cases, a stricture in the urethra can cause the same poor performance.

A pressure-flow study can distinguish a weak bladder muscle from a mechanical obstruction. In this test, the pressure generated within the bladder is measured along with measurement of the flow rate. If the flow rate is poor but the bladder pressure high, it suggests increased resistance as from an enlarged prostate. If the flow is poor and the bladder pressure is low, the problem may not be related to prostatic obstruction at all.

A bladder that has lost its muscle tone because of diabetes, perhaps, or simply through having been overstretched during a long period of urine retention, also gives such a result.

Ultrasound residual measures the amount of urine left in the bladder after urination. A device, like a flashlight, is applied to the skin of the lower abdomen, and there is a computer print-out of an image and amount of the retention. Normally, there should be less than 50 ml of urine left behind in a bladder after urination. A residual of more than 100 ml is considered significant; residuals between 50 ml and 100 ml are in the grey zone and are subject to different interpretations.

THE INTERNATIONAL PROSTATE SYMPTOM SCORE

The International Prostate Symptom Score, commonly known as the IPSS, is a standardized questionnaire. From a battery of questions, seven stood up to statistical analysis. Three of these related to irritative symptoms:

- How often do you have to urinate within two hours of last having passed urine?
- How often do you have an urgent desire to urinate that cannot be postponed?
- How many times must you urinate during the night?

There were then four questions that related to obstructive symptoms:

- How often do you have a weak stream?
- How often do you have to push to urinate?
- How often does the stream stop in mid-flow and need to be pushed to start again?
- How often do you feel you have not totally emptied your bladder?

These seven questions were scored from one to five depending upon their frequency of occurrence during the past month: Less than one in five times (1), less than half the time (2), half the time (3), more than half the time (4), and almost always (5). The numbers for nocturia corresponded to the number of nighttime visits to the bathroom (one to five). The scores were then added up.

I use this simple test often. Scores of seven and under denote mild symptoms, and patients with these are best left untreated. Scores of between eight and nineteen are considered moderate, and patients with these are good candidates for medical management. Scores between twenty and thirty-five are severe, and patients with these may require surgery.

Doctors, including urologists, are much too busy to have patients fill in their IPSS scores in front of them. The questionnaire may be given to patients to fill out while they are in the waiting room. Either that, or they may return with the form filled out on their next visit.

The symptoms score is just a guideline. A patient with a high score may still try his luck with medications, even though some kind of surgery may have been advised, while another with a lower score may opt for surgery because he does not like taking pills for an indefinite period.

I find the IPSS useful because it helps me advise my patients. Some patients tell me that on another day, depending upon their mood, their scores might be different. Curiously, the symptom score does not question degree of urinary dribbling, which many patients find most annoying.

"No matter how long I stand there shaking it, a few drops are sure to stain my shorts," men typically complain.

I advise these patients to place their hand under and behind the scrotum, to lift up, and massage the passage forward. This manoeuvre can lessen the post-void dribble.

Such are the trials and tribulations of the enlarged prostate. Because of our aging society, and until new drugs are developed, our hospitals and clinics are likely to be inundated for a long time to come with men who cannot urinate properly.

4

ENLARGED PROSTATE:
Medical Treatment

Thirty years ago, before the advent of suitable drugs, there was only one treatment for an enlarged prostate – and that was to cut it out! And given that surgical techniques were not as plentiful and sophisticated then as they are today, this could be a painful ordeal. Now, there are many ways to solve problems caused by an enlarged prostate, with a variety of medications. In this, the choices have become bewildering indeed, even to practising urologists.

THE PROSTATE-SHRINKING PILL

In the mid-1980s, when Merck Pharmaceuticals developed a drug it called Proscar (finasteride), which could actually shrink an enlarged prostate, it thought it had solved all enlargement problems. It was counting its windfall too optimistically.

The company knew that twenty- to twenty-five percent of the income of all urologists came from carving channels in enlarged glands in a surgical procedure known as TURP (Trans-Urethral Resection of Prostate), the most frequently performed operation in the U.S. and Canada after cataract extractions.

To address this dilemma, Merck carried out market research. It learned that between fifty-five and sixty percent of all men in North America develop prostate enlargement. Of this population, it discovered that only three percent had surgery, seventeen percent consulted doctors, and an amazing eighty percent did not bother to seek any medical help whatsoever, certain that their urinary problems were just part of the aging process.

Many older men fervently believed nothing could be done for them anyway, or that if they had consulted doctors they would have been forced to accept an unwanted operation.

The potential for Merck's new drug was astronomical. All it had to do to keep urologists happy was to entice some of those men who made up the eighty percent to go to their doctors' offices. Urologists were likely to see more patients and work more, not less.

Actually, long before the Merck market survey, it was recognized that prostate enlargement started in most men after age forty and was present in fifty percent of men in their fifties and eighty percent of men in their eighties. This was determined by pathologists. They had examined the prostates from men of all ages and determined that the disease starts as a nodule in the middle of the gland, in an inner area of the prostate known as the transitional zone. From there it grows by a little over half a gram annually (actually 0.6 ml), gradually compressing the remaining normal prostate tissue, converting it into tissue like the pulp-peel of an orange.

The growth of prostate tissue may not be as regular as I have implied, but more in fits and spurts so that there may be long periods when there is no detectable progression in prostate size at all. Certainly, that is a pattern seen in clinical practice: a man may have an enlarged prostate causing minimal symptoms, and these may remain with him for years. Then, for no apparent reason, there may be symptomatic progression associated with an obvious increase in the size of the gland.

The story of how the Merck scientists created the pill to shrink the prostate has been told many times. A handful of men, possibly inbred, and living in the Dominion Republic, lacked an enzyme from birth called 5-alpha reductase. This enzyme was responsible

28

for converting testosterone into its more powerful form, dihydrotestosterone. When this conversion failed to occur, a boy was born with a sex organ, though external, that made him look more like a girl. His penis was so small, it could be mistaken for a clitoris, his testicles were undescended, and his scrotum so scanty that it resembled labia.

Sometimes, the boys were raised as girls until, at puberty, they developed all the features of the adult male: a normal-sized penis, testicles in the scrotum, and a triangular shaped pubic hair distribution which, pointing to the belly-button, was in distinct contrast to the straight-across female hair distribution. Inside the bodies of these adolescent males, however, the prostate gland did not enlarge.

"What if this enzyme activity were to be blocked in adult life by a simple pill?" the scientists wondered. "Would the prostate gland stop enlarging? Would enlarged prostate glands start shrinking? Could a pill make such a difference?"

Chemists at Merck, however, were not the only ones working toward restricting prostate enlargement. Scientists at Smith Kline Beecham, Glaxo, and other pharmaceutical firms were also hard at work on a solution. Merck simply won the race, that's all, and, in so doing, many thousands of men across the world were able to see considerable improvements in their prostate woes.

How did the pill work? If testosterone is converted to dihydrotestosterone in the presence of the enzyme 5-alpha reductase, how could the enzyme be eliminated?

It was accomplished by eliminating the enzyme's action via a process known as competitive inhibition, that's how. If we make a molecule that has the chemical appearance of testosterone, but doesn't behave like it, the enzyme 5-alpha reductase latches on to it, gets blotted up by it, so to speak, and is thus unavailable to make the conversion it was supposed to carry out – that is, from testosterone to dihydrotestosterone.

When Merck Pharmaceuticals originally asked urologists at McGill University, among many other centres, to conduct Proscar's phase-three studies, the secret drug was called MK-907. It did not take a rocket scientist to figure that MK stood for Merck and 907 stood for the 907th formulation of Proscar that had been tried. Perhaps it was the 900 series in the Merck laboratories and just the 7th formulation tried. The study was double-blind and placebo-controlled. This meant that neither the patient nor the doctor knew who was getting the pill that contained the active drug and who was getting the pill that looked the same but contained no active ingredient.

The drug trial showed that MK-906 did indeed shrink the prostate by about twenty percent in one year, increase the maximum urine flow rate by 3 ml per second after one year, and lower PSA count by forty percent in six months, fifty percent in one year. The twenty-percent shrinkage may not seem like much, but when it occurs where it counts, it can be significant. The maximum flow rate change from 7 to 10 ml a second may be a difference of only 3 ml a second, but this can be the difference between discomfort and comfort.

It has been argued that the drop in PSA reading (forty percent in six months and fifty percent in twelve months) can confuse the diagnosis of cancer, but the argument can be turned around. I have placed some patients on the Merck drug with the understanding that a biopsy would be undertaken if the anticipated PSA drop did not occur. Certainly, it is important to get a PSA reading before starting any patient on the pill.

In the trials, 1, 5, and 10 mg doses were tried. There was little difference between the effects of 1 and 5 mg, and no difference between 5 mg and 10 mg. The company settled on marketing the 5 mg daily dosage. (Subsequently, a 1 mg pill has been put on the market to help bald men grow hair. This is called Propecia.)

Proscar had negative features, too; five percent of those men who took the pill suffered impotence that was reversed when they discarded the medication, and at least as many patients reported diminished erections. Ejaculate volumes dropped dramatically in all of these patients, as much as forty percent, and breast swelling occurred in a few (one to two percent). On the plus side, a number of bald men grew hair, and some men may have been protected from developing prostate cancer.

I recall Proscar being presented at a press conference when the pill was launched in Canada. "This pill may have the same impact Tagamet had on ulcers, eliminating eighty percent of surgery," I said. It was the clip used on television that night.

Although Proscar works well, with results that are maintained for many years, and it continues to be prescribed, sales of it have not lived up to expectations. The pill shrinks very large glands – those over 40 g – but does little for those men who have only slightly enlarged prostates. The smaller glands, however, tend to respond better to another family of drugs called alpha blockers.

THE ALPHA-BLOCKER STORY

If decongestants, or alpha-stimulation, can cause urinary retention, as I have explained, it seems reasonable to expect that alpha-blockers, with exactly the opposite action, can *improve* urinary flow, and they do.

Actually, alpha-blockers have long been on the market as good medications for lowering blood pressure. The pill achieves this by relaxing the muscle cells within the walls of the arteries. In much the same way, it reduces tension in the muscle cells within the prostate gland, thus helping many patients to void better and more comfortably. To those men who take them, and are happy with them, the effect is akin to a faucet that has been opened up a little more to pass more fluid.

The first blood pressure pill in the alpha-blocker family that was used to help men with prostate enlargement was Minipress (prazosin), which was released in 1981. It worked quite well, but had to be taken three times a day, and was highly likely to cause a stuffy nose. Subsequently, in the late 1980s, Hytrin (terazosin) and Cardura (doxazosin) were on the scene. Both were prescribed to be taken in small doses at night, and titrated to a higher effective dose. Five to ten mg of Hytrin or 4 to 8 mg of Cardura are both widely used despite known side effects. Patients who sometimes complain of feeling faint or dizzy are cautioned to move slowly when arising from their beds, especially when they take the pill for the first time.

A more specific alpha-blocker called Flomax (tamsulosin), was approved for release in 1998. Unlike its predecessors, this drug targets muscle cells in the prostate, sphincter, and bladder neck more specifically and does not have as many side effects.

Flomax is promoted as a medication that does not require escalating dosages, nor does it cause dizziness or fainting spells. In Japan, where this drug was developed, it is sold as only a 0.2 mg capsule rather than a 0.4 mg pill as is the case in North America. This suggests that in Japan, where prostatic problems are less common, men can function quite well on smaller doses.

Although Flomax has become a very popular drug, some patients prefer the effects of Hytrin or Cardura, complaining that Flomax made them have a dry ejaculate, yet another side effect. Patients with increased blood pressure may be better off on Hytrin or Cardura anyway, and it will generally cost them less at the pharmacy. Unlike Proscar, the alpha-blockers work almost immediately.

Pills to compete with Flomax have also come into the market. Xatral (alfulosin) works about as well as Flomax, and there is virtually no retrograde ejaculation associated with it. Younger men prefer Xatral because they enjoy the gush associated with ejaculation, while older men often tell me their sex life is less messy with Flomax.

Some time before Hytrin became established as a standard medication for prostate enlargement, I had heard that Dr. Herbert Lepor had been successful with it in the U.S. It was then that I began prescribing it for my patients in Montreal. One day, I received a surprise phone call from someone at Abbott Laboratories, the manufacturer of Hytrin.

"Our sales of this drug have gone up in Montreal," he said, "and we have traced it to you. What's going on? After all, you are not a doctor we associate with hypertension."

I was stunned.

"Hypertension?" I said.

"Yes. Hypertension. This drug is precisely for that."

I had no idea that my prescribing pattern was so easily accessed by pharmaceutical firms. Nor did I think any one would question what I prescribed for which ailment. I regained my composure and said, "Don't you know you have a fantastic pill to help people suffering from prostate enlargement?"

"Really?" said the voice on the line.

"Yes."

The people at Abbott, I said to myself, don't know what a gem they have. I called my stockbroker and placed an order for Abbott stocks. I have done well with that purchase .

Flomax remains a very popular drug to treat men with symptoms of an enlarged prostate. It is also often prescribed with a prostate-shrinking pill, like Proscar .

Both drugs have competition today. Flomax is challenged by Xatral (alfulosin), which is associated with less retrograde or backward ejaculation. A third pill, called Rapaflo (silodosin) has recently been released by Watson Pharmaceuticals. It promises results that are just as good or better. Proscar is challenged by Avodart (dutasteride), which blocks a second chemical reaction, thus making it potentially more powerful.

HERBAL PREPARATIONS

People who promote food additives, herbs, and organic products have bamboozled the public into believing that, unlike the pharmaceutical industry, they have citizens' best interests at heart.

Unfortunately, exactly the opposite may hold true. The pharmaceutical industry may be spectacularly profitable, but at least it comes under stringent government controls. Not so for food additives. Thus, products like saw palmetto are touted as every bit as good as Proscar with none of its side effects, and with only anecdotal evidence and other testimonials as the basis for their claims.

I recommend saw palmetto in my practice, however, because it is non-toxic, and a number of patients have been impressed with its effects on their urination. There is no study, however, that has demonstrated that – like Proscar – it can improve urine flow by 3 ml a second, reduce the size of the prostate by twenty percent, and lower the PSA count by forty percent in six months. Is saw palmetto better than the thirty-percent improvement we can expect from a placebo product? I suspect it might be, but I am not sure.

These remarks about saw palmetto, the best of the herbal preparations, may be applied to pumpkin seed (a good source of vitamin-E, by the way), pygeum, stinging nettle, dwarf palm, and rye, among several other natural substances that can be bought from health stores. I have to admit, however, that I have had no experience with these products.

5

ENLARGED PROSTATE:
Surgical Treatment

When all medications have failed, the urologist has no choice but to try to alleviate the symptoms of a large prostate with surgery. This, I am pleased to tell you, is relatively uncomplicated.

When I first started my training in urology, the operation for an enlarged prostate, which I personally witnessed and helped carry out, was a rather crude two-stage affair. In the first stage, a large rubber pipe about an inch in diameter was inserted, under local anaesthetic, below the belly button and into the bladder. Two weeks later, the patient was wheeled back into the operating room where, under a spinal or general anaesthetic, the pipe was removed.

The surgeon then placed his index finger into the hole the pipe had left, and, after breaking through the urethra, used it to actually gouge out the enlarged prostate tissue. When the index finger could not reach the prostate because the patient had a large belly, toothed forceps were used to tug the offending tissue free.

Surprisingly, hardly any patients bled to death, although transfusions were more frequent in those days than they are today. Although this sounds rather primitive, the happy survival rate accompanying this surgery was testimony to its effectiveness.

I suspect it was the prospect of having to undergo such an operation that kept many patients away from hospitals. It may also have been why so many men minimized their discomforts until they had developed urinary retention. Then they had no choice but to undergo this procedure.

Today, I am pleased to tell you, medical science has progressed beyond this stage; in fact, there are as many surgical procedures for an enlarged prostate as there are prostate-shrinking drugs. The choices of what to do have become bewildering. Furthermore, surgical treatments can be carried out either through the urethra or through the skin.

Some operations are minimally invasive procedures that rely on injections. Others are treatments, as we will discover, that depend on the application of either heat or cold to eliminate excess prostate tissue. So, if you can't cut it out, you may be able to burn it or even freeze it out! Faced with this array of choices, today's urological surgeon earns his stripes both by his skill and by his choices of procedures. No two cases are exactly alike; therefore, the mediated approach has become the gold standard.

Any major procedure in a hospital operating room requires the presence of a surgeon, an assistant (either a colleague doctor or a trainee urologist), an anaesthesiologist, a scrub nurse, and a "floating" or circulating nurse. The surgeon is the acknowledged "star," but he or she can be upstaged accidentally or deliberately by any of the other players. It is not without reason that the operating room is commonly called the theatre, and there can actually be some real-life drama there, too! I should add at this point, that the OR, as it is called, is not necessarily the strict "business-only" environment people feel it to be. Although there is no doubt that the medicine practised there is cool, calm and collected, it is not uncommon to hear anything from classical to rock music in the background. The conversation may range from the surgery itself to politics, humour or any current topic that presents itself. A good surgical team never loses its focus on the patient, but there is a wonderful element of camaraderie, which exists here as well. Now, on to the surgery itself!

Before any kind of prostate surgery, the patient, often groggy from medications that are meant to sedate him and dry his throat, is wheeled from the ward to the operating room where he is placed on a specially designed table under the glare of overhead lamps.

The first specialist who sees him is the anaesthesiologist, and I must tell you that medical treatment is never more intense than when the patient is in the hands of this professional. After all, the anaesthesiologist must ensure that the patient is completely prepared for the first incision. It is no secret that a lot of men I treat are petrified not so much about what I will do to them, but about how they will withstand whatever anaesthesia will be used.

There are three kinds of anaesthesia:

- Spinal
- Epidural
- General

For both kinds of regional anaesthetics, the patient must first sit on the side of the operating table, arching his back by bending over a pillow. This is to permit easier access to a space between lower vertebrae, where the anaesthesiologist's needle will be inserted.

In spinal anaesthesia, an anaesthetic drug like that used by a dentist to block pain is injected into the spinal cord itself. Once the anaesthesiologist has located the spinal fluid, he knows he is in the right place. He then administers the drug.

In epidural anaesthesia, the anaesthetist places a tube into a space outside the spinal cord. Here, with as many repeated doses of an anaesthetic drug as may be necessary, he freezes the nerves, which, if left functioning, would transmit the pain signals to the patient's brain.

When a general anaesthetic is used, the patient is first put to sleep with a drug administered through an intravenous line the anaesthesiologist has inserted in his forearm. This takes effect in a matter of seconds. Then a drug to paralyse all muscles is administered into the same line, and a tube is inserted into his windpipe to prevent him from swallowing his tongue.

It is through this endo-tracheal tube that the patient is ventilated and kept anaesthetized with sleep-inducing gases, such as ether or chloroform. In recent years, however, these agents have been replaced by newer, better, and safer drugs.

Blood pressure and heartbeat are monitored continuously throughout all prostate surgeries. In potentially complicated – and bloody – cases, a needle will be inserted into an artery in the wrist so that the patient's oxygen level in the arterial blood can be monitored. Another thin plastic tube may be inserted into the jugular vein so that the pressure in veins near the heart can be measured. This measurement helps the anaesthesiologist decide if blood and fluid replacements during the operation are adequate, or whether they need to be increased.

While the anaesthetic is being prepared, the circulating nurse ascertains that all the instruments and supplies are ready for the urologist to begin the operation. She also helps the scrub nurse keep an accurate count of the sponges, needles, and instruments used.

Like the surgeon, the scrub nurse is scrubbed, gowned, and gloved. It is her duty to pass various instruments to the surgeon as he goes about his job. A good scrub nurse will anticipate the surgeon's needs and have the appropriate instrument in his hands almost before he asks for it.

It is difficult to imagine an operating room procedure today without thinking of a lot of scrubbing of hands and arms, and various, sometimes multicoloured head coverings, gowns, boots, and gloves. Surgical gloves, however, were introduced only a century ago. Dr. William Halstead, a prominent American surgeon, provided the first pair of these for his nurse because she had a skin condition and couldn't otherwise participate, and Dr. Halstead needed her help.

The operation starts with the surgeon, and/or his or her assistant, standing on opposite sides of the operating table applying an antiseptic paint such as iodine to the area where the skin must be cut. Sterile drapes cover the patient from head to toe except for that part of his body that must be exposed.

Today, surgery is routinely applied for extremely large prostates. That is to say, those over 200 g. For this procedure, I usually make a lateral incision – a "bikini cut," it's called – one centimetre above the pubic bone. I then prise apart the recti muscles that run the length of the torso, so I can view the frontal surface of the prostate gland. After that, I make a transverse cut over the prostate capsule, and, with my index finger, simply gouge out – or enucleate – the enlarged tissue. In other words, my finger finds the plane between the enlarged gland and the capsule formed by normal tissue that has been compressed by unwanted tissue. It's a bit like removing the fruit of a tangerine after the peel has been cut, and is often just as easy.

This procedure is called a retropubic prostatectomy and was first introduced by the British surgeon, Terrence Millan, in 1947. The operation became established in the 1960s, and remains a commonly performed procedure, although it is being challenged today by the Holmoum laser enucleation procedure.

I performed a retropubic prostatectomy on a sixty-four-year-old semi-retired businessman who weighed 248 pounds, stood five feet ten inches tall, and who had denied, minimized, even ignored his health care issues until he passed a very bloody urine specimen. At this point he had had no choice but to consult his family doctor, who arranged an abdominal ultrasound examination. This revealed a solid lump measuring 6.5 cm long in his left kidney, an enlarged prostate gland, and four stones in his bladder, each the size of a robin's egg.

Any one of this man's three disorders could have been responsible for his bloody urine. A CT scan (Computerized Tomogram) confirmed the presence of kidney cancer, but showed no evidence that the disease had spread into the veins that carry blood out of the kidneys, or into the lymph nodes. A trans-rectal ultrasound assessment of the man's prostate gland, however, revealed it to be the size of a baseball, and weighing 212 g.

I proposed placing the patient on his side, removing his cancerous kidney, and then, if all was well, re-positioning him on his back for a retropubic prostatectomy and then the removal of the bladder stones through the same opening of the prostatic capsule. I warned the patient that his excess weight put him at extra risk for wound infection, pneumonia, and phlebitis.

The three-in-one operation went smoothly, and his post-operative course was uneventful. The patient was so pleased with the outcome that he promised to submit to regular medical check-ups in the future.

Consider, too, a sixty-six-year-old retired professor who, on rectal examination, displayed a very large, soft prostate, and who had clear urine that was nicely free of red and white blood cells. His very large gland and urine-flow difficulties had suggested a need for immediate surgical correction, but this patient wanted to give a medical approach a longer trial, and I agreed, recognizing that his woes were quite routine.

For one year, the retired professor had taken the alpha-blocker Cardura in 4 mg doses and Proscar in 5 mg doses. His PSA count had now dropped from 12.0 to 5.8. An ultrasound examination showed that the prostate was calculated to weigh 140 g, with no images that might suggest cancer. His improvement had been light, but, as he intended to travel extensively in the coming years, he finally took my advice and underwent a retropubic prostatectomy. 82 g of tissue was removed. Today, this man is pleased that he decided not to postpone the surgery any longer.

TRANS-URETHRAL RESECTION OF THE PROSTATE – THE TURP

While the retropubic prostatectomy is a neat procedure with a predictable outcome, it has been challenged in popularity by what is called a TURP. This is the most common surgical procedure of all for an enlarged prostate. TURPs are now so popular among both doctors and their patients that, at the height of my career, I performed a hundred of them annually, almost always with positive results.

The operation itself is really quite simple. After the anaesthetic has been administered – this can be either general or spinal – the patient is placed in stirrups, assuming the position of a woman about to deliver a baby. The genital area is then washed with an antiseptic solution, and the legs and lower abdomen are draped with a sterile covering.

TRANS-URETHRAL RESECTION OF THE PROSTATE (TURP)

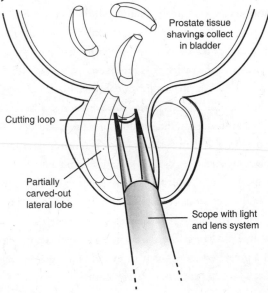

Prostate tissue shavings collect in bladder

Cutting loop

Partially carved-out lateral lobe

Scope with light and lens system

The urethra is lubricated and dilated to accept a long metal pipe called a resectoscope (a variation on the cystoscope), which is about a centimetre in diameter. It is fitted with a fibre-optic light that illuminates the passage and an electrical current powerful enough to function as a scalpel. The resectoscope is passed through the tip of the penis and eased through the urethra into the bladder.

During the operation, the electrically activated wire loop is drawn back and forth rather like a crocheting hook. With many short excursions of the loop – always from the farthest point to the nearest – the obstructing prostate tissue is neatly carved away. If arterial spurts are seen, as they often are, the bleeding can be stopped by switching the foot pedal, like using the brake instead of the accelerator. This changes the nature of the current in the wire loop from one that cuts to one that cauterizes blood vessels.

When the resection has been completed, the tissue chips are flushed out of the bladder, and a special Foley catheter is inserted to provide continuous irrigation. A smaller in-flow channel allows a saline solution to wash out the bladder, and a larger out-flow channel drains out the wash, which invariably contains some blood. When the drainage is largely blood-free, the in-flow is stopped, and within a day or so the catheter is removed.

Patients usually urinate quite comfortably one day after a TURP, though there is sometimes some burning. The usual blood loss from the procedure is under 500 ml – a mere cupful – but about the same amount is lost after the operation as during it. Blood transfusions are sometimes necessary, but are not routine.

Some measure of the surgeon's skill is reflected in the size of the prostate he decides to tackle, and sometimes pride overrides prudence. A good urological surgeon can carve out 60 g. of obstructing tissue in less than an hour. Some experienced urologists can deal with a prostate that is not too severely enlarged within forty-five minutes. If the operation lasts two hours, however, it is usually

42

far too long for comfort: Prolonged scratching by the resectoscope on the urinary lining can lead to scarring of the urethra. Such scarring causes a narrowing of the passage called a stricture, and this may necessitate surgical correction in the future. Today, TURPs can be performed with the surgeons watching their work on a television screen instead of looking directly through their resectoscope lenses. In this way, the operation can be done with higher magnification and without the surgeon having to contort his head and neck as he carves a passage through the tissue. Teaching the procedure has also become easier, because the teacher can interrupt the trainee at any point. Surgical accidents have become much less frequent as a consequence. Nevertheless, older urologists – those who are generally used to employing the traditional method – sometimes feel more comfortable with what has worked so successfully for them in the past .

Whatever the method used, urologists aim to send all their patients home within a day or two after their TURPs. It is a kind of success rate that comes with years of urological experience, and sometimes with an inborn talent.

WHEN THINGS GO WRONG

The ideal TURP – 60 g of tissue pared away in sixty minutes – is not always achieved without complications. Sometimes, for instance, even when the surgeon feels he has succeeding in limiting bleeding during the operation, the patient may begin to lose a lot of blood in the recovery room afterwards.

Such was the case of a sixty-five-year-old school teacher who had had a routine TURP that went very well. When his bleeding worsened, I sought to slow it down simply by making the fluid that was irrigating the bladder – routinely at room temperature – ice cold. Fresh bleeding persisted, however. Clots formed within the bladder that could not be evacuated. Six hours after his TURP, the patient had to be taken back into the operating room.

There, copious clots in the bladder were evacuated with a syringe, but I could not discern where the bleeding had actually started. A rigid catheter known as a haematuric catheter that allows more vigorous irrigation was placed through the man's urethra into his bladder, and he was returned to the recovery room. There was no further bleeding, I am happy to say, and the recovery was normal after that.

What I have described here is not common, but not so unusual, either. Sometimes persistent bleeding during or after a TURP occurs because the irrigation solution was inadvertently allowed to run dry. The speed of irrigation is determined by the amount of bleeding; when bleeding is brisk, the irrigation must be rapid – almost a flow rather than a mere drip. Under these circumstances, a three-litre irrigation bag can be used up quickly, and if it is not immediately replaced, clots can fill the bladder.

Sometimes, the irrigation is as slow as an intravenous drip. Even then, if the nurse attending the patient does not replace an irrigation bag that has run dry, there can be problems with clot retention. There are times when a bleeding point has been insufficiently cauterized. At other times, an artery that has been in spasm and had appeared to be controlled suddenly begins to bleed.

Such surgical setbacks can occur even when the patient is in the best of hands, but they are more frequent when a novice surgeon tackles too large a gland. Problems most often arise when the carving-out process has been too deep in some places – too aggressive near the bladder neck, for example, thus creating a nasty perforation – or too shallow in others.

When the resection is too shallow, the prostate tissue left behind falls into the cavity, obstructing the urinary passage, and there is no relief of symptoms. This can be corrected with a second procedure. Fortunately, unlike operations that require an incision, a previous TURP does not make a redo more difficult, because there is no extra scar tissue en route with which to contend.

When the cut is too deep, the prostate wall can be perforated. This may allow the irrigating fluid the surgeon has been using to accumulate in the tissue outside the urinary tract. At this point, the operation must be aborted because the abdomen will swell, and the patient will need a separate drainage procedure or time – usually a couple of days – to absorb the fluid naturally.

One patient who suffered this setback complained of severe pain beyond the control of his spinal anaesthetic – before the operation was completed. His abdomen began to swell enormously and became rigid. The procedure was halted, and the bleeding was stopped by the insertion of a catheter – complete with balloon which, when fully inflated, was able to plug the bleeding in the lower bladder. The man's intestines remained paralysed for a few days, but slowly recovered. No further surgery was necessary. The patient is grateful he survived the ordeal and could urinate comfortably without more operations.

This second complication can be more critical. It is possible for unwanted irrigating fluid to actually enter large veins in the prostate area. This fluid contains a protein that simulates body fluid, but because it lacks salt, it will not conduct the electricity the surgeon needs for his resectoscope during the operation. Not only that, but when large amounts of this fluid are absorbed into the bloodstream, the sodium becomes depressed while the volume of water increases. The result of this is a form of water poisoning. The patient becomes confused, agitated, even temporarily blinded and comatose – a condition known as "TURP syndrome."

One such patient was a man of eighty-six. He had no medical history of serious health problems and, despite his age, was not considered a high-risk TURP candidate. The procedure was uneventful until it was almost complete, at which point the man became agitated and nauseous, and retched. The anaesthesiologist reported a rise in his blood pressure and asked me if he might be absorbing fluid. It was indeed possible. A few moments were taken to assure adequate control of all bleeding, and I terminated the operation immediately. Later, in the intensive care unit, the patient complained of blurred vision, then loss of vision. Usually, unless a patient in this condition is treated promptly, with strong diuretics (water pills) and intravenous infusions of concentrated saline, he may die.

Fortunately, this one needed neither. In fact, the statistics were on his side. While one in a hundred TURP patients may suffer this complication, few will succumb to it. In fact, in my entire career, I have never ever witnessed a TURP syndrome fatality.

I have taught a generation of resident doctors how to perform this operation, and it continues to fascinate me why some of them struggle endlessly to master it, while others do so with an economy of effort and style. I suspect it is like learning to accomplish reasonable heights in a sport. When it comes to manual dexterity and the perception of three-dimensional configurations, some people are simply more gifted than others. Both of these attributes are needed to restore a prostate to its normal function.

SIDE EFFECTS

A disconcerting side effect of the TURP is what is known as the "dry" ejaculation. There is ejaculation, in fact, except that now the semen is discharged into the bladder instead externally. This is neither dangerous nor a cause for alarm. It is a problem only to those patients who intend to father another child. In no way does it diminish the intensity of the orgasm.

While many patients confess to being unhappy about the dry ejaculation, some actually prefer sex that's "less messy."

More serious is the fact that twenty-five percent of patients who have had a TURP report diminished erections. Some say they have not been able to get an erection at all since surgery.

There is no good explanation for either of these conditions. Could the nerves have been damaged by the electrical current? This does not seem likely, unless the carving process was extended beyond the confines of the prostate. More probable is this: patients are much more likely to blame the surgical assault for their erectile dysfunctions and forget how imperfectly they may have performed before it.

A much more likely explanation then is that the blood flow to the penis in older men is usually weaker than it once was — just as it may be somewhat diminished to the heart or brain.

MINIMALLY INVASIVE PROCEDURES

Complications with the TURP have encouraged a search for easier and simpler ways to manage enlarged prostate problems than having to undergo surgery.

Balloon dilatation may have been the first of the simple substitutes. A Foley catheter was adapted so that upon filling its little balloon, it would distend the prostatic urethra that was obstructed by the enlarged gland. The idea was borrowed from the angioplasty for arteriosclerotic coronary arteries. The cholesterol plaques can be compressed like snowflakes, but prostatic tissue behaves more like shifting sand.

Temporary relief lasting weeks, even up to a month or two, could be achieved by balloon dilation, but the results were much too short to justify the anaesthetic involved. So the procedure was abandoned.

A second less-invasive method works very well for urethral strictures. It uses a scaffold-like contraption called a stent, which is made of titanium. This is like a short length of wire used to contain chickens that has been miniaturized and rolled into a cylindrical shape. When placed though a scarred urethra, the spring in the mesh distends the coil to a wider diameter, thus enlarging the opening. The titanium is inert to tissue reaction, and, within a matter of weeks, the "mesh" is overgrown by normal tissue.

The same coil can be placed through the prostatic urethra to keep the obstructing prostatic tissue from caving in. If the length of the coil is just right, it can work. If, however, the coil extends beyond the prostate gland, there can be problems. Stones may form on a section that reaches into the bladder, and a length that extends distally beyond the prostate will prevent the sphincter from functioning, rendering the patient incontinent.

With accurate placement of the device and improved design, a role may be still found for the titanium-wall stent in the management of enlarged prostates.

THERMAL THERAPY

Heat and cold, and fire and ice, are not new. Government agencies like the Health Protection Branch in Canada and the Food and Drug Administration in the U.S., have no jurisdiction over medical devices that utilize extreme temperatures, yet temperature has been part of our lives since time immemorial, and temperature is used to alleviate many prostate problems.

There are risks that hot-cold devices may, if government is not involved, be promoted with very little scientific validation. By the same token, honest efforts to invent and promote such devices may fail to get appropriate attention.

Devices that are used to raise the prostate temperature to 40 degrees centigrade do very little to the gland and yet are promoted to help people with prostatic symptoms. Just as a sauna makes a patient feel better, heat treatment may help alleviate a man's symptoms. There will, however, be no change in the size of his gland, nor any improvement in the flow of his urine.

Devices that raise the temperature of the prostate to 60 degrees centrigrade are useful because they can destroy live prostate tissue, which leads to some sloughing and a consequent reduction in the gland's size. There may be a place for such treatment, but it is not appropriate for the severely enlarged prostate.

Other surgical ways to treat an enlarged prostate include TUNA, or Trans-Urethral Needle Ablation, which uses radio-frequency energy to punch holes in the prostate. This results in lessening the resistance to urine flow, and is easily tolerated by patients. Its effectiveness, however, is less certain.

Whenever I suggest any kind of surgery, patients will ask if I will use the laser. When I say no, they are invariably disappointed. They were hoping that a "magic wand" would be used.

"Would you use a blow torch to light candles on a birthday cake?" I ask. When they look at me as if to say, "Why not?" I interject, "You wouldn't use a power saw to cut a match-stick, would you?"

Laser energy does have multiple uses in urological surgery, though. It has proven useful for superficial tumours of the bladder, for breaking up stones in the ureters and bladder, and for reducing prostate size by vaporization, that is to say, eliminating tissue that obstructs urine.

The first lasers for handling prostate enlargement shot beams into the prostate that had been reflected, by a mirror, at a right angles. They killed tissue for varying depths and widths, depending upon the amount of energy used. The dead tissue then sloughed and was voided out over a period of several months. Dead tissue that was not washed out on urination, however, often obstructed the flow, and a catheter had to be left in place for several months at a time. Nonetheless, patients did not bleed, and for some patients this was a worthwhile treatment.

An example of such a patient could be someone on anti-coagulation therapy or one for whom temporary interruption of these blood thinners might be dangerous – a patient who has suffered a recent heart attack, for instance, and has been prescribed Coumadin.

Laser energy using holmium can also be used. This makes *direct* contact with the prostate and vaporizes tissue instantly. Holmium lasers can carve out large glands without any significant blood loss. In effect, they remove prostate tissue in much the same way that my finger enucleates the gland in a retropubic prostatectomy. The laser tip finds the plane between the enlarged tissue and the compressed tissue that has formed the false capsule of the gland. The enucleated gland is then left to float freely inside the bladder.

At this point, another instrument called a morsellator, which can be likened to a meat grinder fitted with a vacuum cleaner, reduces the tissue to a pulp and sucks it out. It is then strained and submitted for pathological examination.

The holmium laser is an improvement over previous laser techniques and will find its place among all the treatment options available. The holmium laser enucleation of very large prostates, those over 100 g, challenges the traditional retropubic prostatectomy. The hospitalization is significantly shorter, one day versus a few days. But the learning curve for the procedure is much longer and, even in experienced hands, the procedure is time-consuming, taking three hours over one hour for the open procedure. Operating room access, more than anything else, has limited its wide-scale adoption.

Microwave energy is also being used to ablate prostate tissue. This procedure is called TUMT – Transurethral Microwave Thermal Therapy. The microwave is generated by a device called a Prostatron, which is placed in the rectum. The heat it emits is captured by an antenna placed in the urethral catheter, and this heats the gland to a temperature of between 60 and 75 degrees centigrade, killing unwanted tissue, which sloughs out over a period of weeks.

HIFU is the acronym for High Intensity Focused Ultrasound. Here, ultrasound energy is focused precisely to produce comparable amounts of heat that can destroy prostate tissue.

Prostate tissue can also be destroyed by cooling the gland to a temperature close to freezing. This technique is being tried more to eradicate cancerous tissue than to eliminate unwanted tissue, but the principle remains much the same as that used in heat treatments.

After all this you might think these different techniques represent totally different modalities of treatment. In fact, they just represent different ways of using hot and cold.

Cold can freeze the prostate and cause frozen tissue to be sloughed, but heat is generally more effective. Its use is akin to burning a hole through a block of wood by applying a red hot branding iron to it, burning a hole by firing a blow torch, or creating a hole by concentrating the rays of the sun with a magnifying glass.

Yet another way to obliterate prostate tissue is to eradicate it by injecting chemicals directly into the gland. Pure alcohol can be used in this way, and it is both reasonably effective and very inexpensive. Promising results from this novel approach are just beginning to be reported. In the final analysis, however, an experienced surgeon can carve out obstructing tissue more completely, more precisely, and more effectively than any heat-generating or cold-generating devices available, although holmium laser experts may challenge me on this point.

SURGICAL STUDIES

Surprisingly, worldwide urological studies carried out first in Denmark and then across the world throughout the 1970s and 1980s revealed that serious consequences, such as cardiac deaths in extreme cases, were more frequent with TURPs than they were with procedures that involved incisions.

How could this be? How could a procedure that eliminates a surgical incision – and could therefore be considered less taxing on the body – be associated with such severe problems?

The urological community was shocked by these findings, and many centres began to re-examine their own results. Was it actually true that patients undergoing TURPs were more likely to have a cardiac death soon after surgery than those who had prostatectomies with an incision? And was it also correct that patients needed to return for second TURPs because of the re-growth of tissue more often than if they had undergone retropubic prostatectomies? By and large, these findings were confirmed.

At the University of Manitoba, a careful analysis carried out by Dr. Ernest Ramsey also supported these results. He reported that thirteen percent of patients who had undergone a TURP required a repeat procedure. This compared with only four percent of those who had had an open prostatectomy.

Dr. Ramsey also maintained that the death rate among patients five years after TURPs was higher than among those who had undergone the open procedure. He discovered, however, that sicker patients were generally directed towards TURPs rather than open procedures, because the former would be less traumatic for them. This meant that the deaths of these patients may not have been exclusively due to the effects of their TURPs, but from other factors.

6

ENLARGED PROSTATE:
Mimicking Disorders

Many symptoms attributed to an enlarged prostate may not be due to this annoying condition at all. A scar in the urethra that has been caused by an infection – specifically gonorrhoea – can create the same obstruction. Such scarring, however, is much more likely to be the result of an instrument having been passed through the urethra than by a sexually transmitted infection.

Urethral strictures are very often caused by simple catheterization, a routine procedure that can be damaging when it has not been done with adequate lubrication. The guilty parties here are often emergency room staffers who should know better, but who are under time constraints and have a limited knowledge of urology. To be fair, urethral strictures can sometimes be the result of scarring following the rough passage of a cystoscope or resectoscope in the urology department itself!

A stone in the bladder that is small enough to pass into the urethra will also impede urine flow and create a blockage that suggests an enlarged prostate.

Other mimicking symptoms are due to irritations rather than an obstruction. Patients who have these feel the same effects – the need to urinate frequently and urgently, both day and night. Diseases and disorders that create these annoying symptoms include Parkinson's disease, strokes, spinal stenosis, and multiple sclerosis. That is to say, any disturbance to the brain or spinal canal will disturb messages informing the bladder it does not yet have to contract.

Before telling you why prostate symptoms occur with these seemingly unrelated disorders, I would like to explain how the bladder works, and how urination ideally occurs.

Make no mistake about it, the bladder is a marvel in engineering design. When I lecture my medical students I talk about how this fine mechanism functions in normal life and how it can be disturbed by different medical disorders. I usually start by telling them how the bladder gets short shrift in medical school teaching because it is "a non-vital organ," one that is considered unnecessary for comfortable living – a kind of tank, if you like, that has been installed in the pelvic region simply to collect liquid waste. How unfair!

The kidney, on the other hand, receives a lot of time and attention because it appears to have a more important function. By producing large or small volumes of urine, the kidney is able to render the body either drier or moister. Also, by changing the acidity of the urine, it can make the body more acid or more alkaline. In other words, the kidney is responsible for maintaining the body's healthy levels of acidity and liquidity while filtering unwanted fluid – urine – into the bladder.

Doctors like to manipulate, or fine-tune, the functions of the kidney by prescribing drugs likes diuretics. These are "water pills" that essentially dry out the body by making a person produce more urine. On the other hand, doctors may advise a patient to add baking soda to a glass of water as an ongoing treatment for excess acidity. Rendering the urine more alkaline can dissolve a uric acid stone, but it may take weeks to months to achieve this objective.

They may even tell a patient who has a history of kidney failure – uraemia – to consume less protein so as to make fewer demands on the kidneys. Uraemia, we must remember, occurs when the body cannot eliminate the end products of protein and cannot control acidity or fluidity. This may lead to other distressing ailments.

I tell my students, however, that for all its importance, the work of the kidney can be replaced by a simple sheet of cellophane, and they raise their eyebrows.

Why? How?

A sheet of simple household cellophane is the essential component of the artificial kidney. As a semi-permeable membrane, it can actually strain the blood. As small molecules are able to pass through the pores of the cellophane membrane, the blood-fluid and bath-fluid equilibrate, and the waste products that have accumulated are washed out like dirt from clothing into the water in a washing machine.

You will see from this analogy that it is not too difficult to create an artificial kidney that can function outside the body for people on dialysis. To replace the bladder, though, would be next to impossible. The bladder, after all, requires a morass of nerve endings that tell us when it is time to urinate. Meanwhile, bladder muscles enable us to actually do so – to enjoy this bodily function naturally and fully.

If my lecture were a session with aspiring engineers, I tell my medical students, and I were to ask them to design a mechanical organ that had the properties of the human bladder, a mighty challenge would be in the offing. Engineers would need to create a receptacle that could hold liquid without it leaking, and yet, as it filled, develop absolutely no tension in its wall. Near its capacity, the receptacle would also need to transmit a signal while still continuing to fill, now with a minimal increase in wall pressure. On command, the pressure in the wall of this receptacle would ideally increase, causing it to contract and evacuate its content.

This, in essence, is how a healthy bladder functions. As it fills, it needs to have the properties of an ordinary plastic bag; then, at capacity, it needs to transform itself into a muscular balloon that would literally thrust out the urine. If such a receptacle were made of plastic or metal, the task of urinating on the brain's command would be impossible. The engineers' "bladder" would have to have a faucet. By this reckoning, the human bladder operates as a miracle of anatomy.

How does it do its wonderful work?

The bladder muscles have a unique property, which is called "accommodation." This word is used to define how the muscle fibres in the bladder stretch, then relax automatically, to accommodate an increased volume of urine without an increase in muscle tone.

When the bladder is almost full, there is a mild contraction of these same muscles, which signals the sensation of fullness. The bladder muscles, however, can continue to stretch. Finally, upon voluntary command, they contract to evacuate the bladder's content out through the prostate and the urethra.

This final contraction is rather like the human knee-jerk reflex – stimulate the tendon below the kneecap with a rubber hammer and cause the leg to kick up as the quadriceps, or the thigh muscles, contract. The reaction of the full bladder is like the tap below the kneecap, and the response to this is the contraction of the bladder muscles.

In a healthy person, this function is unconscious. It happens without a need to think about it. The bladder's reflex arc is connected to the brain by nerve fibres that travel up and down in what is called the autonomic nervous system, namely, the sympathetic and parasympathetic nervous system. This system, as I have indicated, is considered involuntary and automatic.

But is it? We do have control of our bladder and bowel; it is not totally involuntary. This misperception of the autonomic nervous system is, in my estimation, a Western phenomenon. Eastern philosophies, like Transcendental meditation, Yoga, Zen, etc, teach that we can control the so-called involuntary nervous system. We can learn to lower the blood pressure, learn to slow the heartbeat, learn to suspend animation, just as we learn to control urination.

And when urination is disturbed, we should be able to retrain the system to behave better. In the West, though, we are more likely to resort to medications.

Patients who suffer from Parkinson's disease, a stroke, a brain tumour, multiple sclerosis, and spinal stenosis urinate with increased frequency. These ailments destroy, disturb, damage, or blunt messages from the brain that normally tell the bladder not to contract. Without these proper "instructions," patients feel many more bladder contractions than normal – "uninhibited" contractions, as they are called in urology – often with nasty effects. In severe cases, the messages are so distorted that patients are unable to hold their urine at all.

This is why patients who suffer from these ailments are all too often referred to urologists for prostate assessment when, in fact, they have no prostate disorders at all.

A patient suffering from congestive heart failure has a slightly different problem. His body will reabsorb the fluid that accumulates in his legs during the day, and this extra fluid, which has made his ankles swell, is voided out with greater-than-normal regularity. Again, the need to urinate often during the night has nothing to do with the prostate gland, but with an excess amount of water in the body.

Diabetes affects nerve endings at many levels. The sensation of bladder filling is less pronounced, consequently the bladder is often distended and rendered atonic – like an un-burst but overstretched balloon.

Stones also cause extra irritation in the bladder wall, increasing the frequency and urgency to void.

Such reasons for disturbed urination patterns must be considered before assuming that prostate enlargement is the reason for the problem. Patients with the earliest symptoms of an enlarged prostate invariably complain of a frequent need to void in the morning – upon rising, for example, then ten minutes later, and again within an hour. After that, the urinary pattern becomes quite normal. How can I explain this? I can't. Not everything in medicine can be accounted for. I can, however, reassure patients that this is a common pattern.

Finally, a simple urine or bladder infection can make urination impossible, sometimes for two or three days at a time. This condition is usually dealt with quite simply with any one of several antibiotics, like Septra (sulphamethoxazole-trimethoprim) or Cipro (ciprofloxacin).

But remember: no one should ever take a urine infection too lightly, because it nearly always means that, for a variety of reasons which need to be accurately diagnosed, the prostate is not allowing the urine to pass freely. In other words, a urine infection may mean that the prostate is functioning as it should.

Stay with me, because we will discover other symptoms that mimic an enlarged prostate – perhaps the human male's most common health problem – when we discuss inflammation of the prostate and various other urological infections.

7

ENLARGED PROSTATE:
Don't Ignore your Symptoms

Of all the factors that might affect a patient's prostate health, there is no doubt that fear ranks among the most powerful. The "ostrich" approach of burying one's head in the proverbial sand and ignoring evident symptoms has led to more illness and death than most others. There is a natural reluctance to go to a doctor and to have your most private parts meticulously examined, with some degree of discomfort involved. For many men, the "It will go away on its own," or the "I really DO feel better today," is the philosophy of choice.

No course of action could be further from the healing truth; in fact, the sooner a man reports his symptoms to his physician, the sooner he will most probably be cured of his problems – in most cases, for the balance of his life.

Chances are that if you are older than fifty, enlarged prostate problems will figure adversely on your well-being, particularly if they run in your family. For this reason alone, you should get both an annual rectal examination and a PSA blood test in a determined effort to ensure that if your prostate is invaded by cancer, you and your doctor will know about it early.

Once the combination of the rectal examination and the PSA have ruled out the likelihood of cancer, the emphasis should then be placed solely on dealing with enlargement issues. The important thing is this, though: don't ignore any symptoms you may have.

When a patient chooses to overlook an enlarged prostate, his medical problems can move in several ways, almost all of them unpleasant.

First, he can develop a sudden and total inability to empty his bladder, a condition known as acute urinary retention, one of the most painful ordeals a man can face. If he is catheterized promptly and agrees to one of the several surgical options available, he should make a complete recovery. If, however, he is unfit for surgery – being within six months of a heart attack, for example, or having recently undergone a major operation – he might be temporarily helped by an indwelling Foley catheter that is changed every month.

On the other hand, his bladder might benefit from being drained through a catheter that is placed through his abdomen until such time as he can have corrective surgery. This procedure is called suprapubic drainage, and, because the catheter does not traverse the length of the urethra and through the prostate, is generally considered safer for the patient because it avoids urethral strictures.

If I had to wear a catheter and a leg bag for a protracted period – more than two months, say – I would insist upon the suprapubic type. If I had a problem with incontinence, however, I might have no choice in the matter.

If a patient's urine retention is not immediately relieved, his bladder will not burst, but he will develop other problems. One of these will be the trickling of urine from the tip of his penis in what is called "overflow" incontinence.

Should that same patient suffer a stomach blow during this time, like a steering wheel injury, his distended bladder could burst internally, spilling urine into his abdominal cavity and causing a severe infection rather like a burst appendix. Without emergency intervention, the outcome could be fatal.

I recall such a case in my first year of urological training. A well-to-do business man had too much liquor before he retired to bed. When he fell out of bed, he had severe abdominal pains and was rushed to hospital. In the Emergency Room, a ruptured bladder was diagnosed. He was taken to the operating room and the rupture repaired. The following morning I described the case to a senior urologist.

"You found a linear tear at the dome," he said.

"Yes, how did you know that?" I asked.

"That's where it always occurs," he said.

"Why?" I persisted.

He ignored me as if to say, "Don't ask any stupid questions."

Subsequently, I blew up bladders of fresh cadavers and observed that the tear was always at the dome. When I repeated the experiment on bladders that had been removed from the cadavers, the tears occurred at random, which proved that support rather than intrinsic weakness determined the site of the tear. This was my first publication in the urological literature.

When the bladder cannot expel urine easily, it will first develop changes to compensate for the increased resistance – a thickening of its wall. To put it simply, the overworked bladder muscles will thicken, just as biceps enlarge with weight-lifting exercises.

Following this, there is a process of de-compensation – what we urologists call a "blowout" from the bladder wall. This, a distortion that resembles a sort of secondary bladder, is called a cellule when small and a diverticulum when large. Of course, there can be cellules or diverticula. The main problem is that a blowout, large or small, is not covered with a layer of muscle and does not therefore empty when the bladder evacuates. Thus, it remains indefinitely as a "bag" of urine, and, in some cases, stones will form within it.

The effects can be quite serious. Incomplete emptying of the bladder exposes the patient to many urinary infections.

This brings us to another course a patient's health may take if he ignores treatment for his enlarged prostate: a gradual deterioration of his kidneys, which is potentially a more serious condition.

Again, a thickening of the bladder muscles is responsible. This can be seen when the attending urologist examines the bladder during a cystoscopy. The crisscrossing muscles that make up the substance of the bladder, he notes, will give the lining a honeycombed appearance called trabeculation. This thickening causes a lengthening of the ureters, and these become tortuous and distended.

More serious is that where they actually enter the bladder, the ureters will be twisted into a fish-hook distortion that will cause the urine to back up.

Suffice it to say that patients who neglect to have these changes treated can eventually experience back-up pressure damage to their kidneys, for which the only treatment may be dialysis.

Unfortunately, patients in this advanced stage still seek treatment, although in developed countries, where medical diagnostics have been greatly improved, they are becoming less and less frequent. Forty years ago, however, they were as common as the two-stage prostatectomy, now as obsolete as the horse and buggy.

MONITORING YOUR SYMPTOMS

My advice is to start keeping a record of your own symptom scores – those lifestyle questions we call the IPSS – to see how they fluctuate, as they surely will. Consider IPSS readings as a guide and nothing more, however, and do not get alarmed if you have a score that has increased over the years because this may be associated with the simple aging process.

Generally speaking, if your IPSS score is seven or less, your urologist will probably decide to do nothing other than monitor your condition lest it should worsen. If is between eight and seventeen you may need medical treatment. If your score is higher that seventeen you may need surgery.

Do not be shy to give alpha-blockers a try to help you urinate a little better — at any stage of your treatment or waiting period. Starting to take these pills does not mean you will have to rely on them forever. If you tend to have high blood pressure, you might ask your doctor if you may try Cardura or Hytrin. If you have a normal or lower than normal blood pressure, use Flomax, Xatral or Rapaflo.

When we stop and think about it, an enlarged prostate constitutes what I like to call a plumbing problem that must be fixed so that the waste water will flow away. It is therefore wise to deal with it before it becomes a major issue that could affect kidney function.

It is debatable whether a change in diet or lifestyle can make any real difference to an ailing prostate once it has started to malfunction. It is possible that diet might have prevented the enlargement in the first place, although this has not been conclusively established, either. More certain is that some diets and off-the-shelf medications have enjoyed some success in helping to alleviate prostate problems.

An innocuous herbal product called saw palmetto, which is derived from a small palm-like tree and which is available in most health food stores, has been known to diminish prostate enlargement symptoms — I repeat, *only the symptoms* and not the enlargement itself. Saw palmetto has fewer side effects than Proscar because it is not nearly as powerful — and not nearly as effective.

Too many off-the-shelf cold products have been known to aggravate prostate obstructions. I talk specifically, of course, about those decongestant remedies. If you catch a cold while you are experiencing voiding difficulties, it would be better if you used either Aspirin or Tylenol.

The prescription drug Proscar or Avodart, meanwhile, is worthwhile if an ultrasound examination has determined that your prostate weighs more than 40 g and is causing symptoms. You should always ask your doctor for a PSA reading before starting one of these drugs so you will see your symptoms improve — and your IPSS score drop.

Many of my patients take both Proscar or Avodart and alpha-blockers to promote urination. I usually start these men on the alpha-blockers and then add Proscar or Avodart if the gland is well over 40 g.

If your prostate is large enough – and annoying enough – don't be afraid of a TURP. In the hands of almost all surgeons, the results are excellent. Don't be afraid, either, of that inevitable side effect. Some men are actually quite grateful for internal ejaculation, particularly those who no longer want to father children .

Be prepared to listen to other options that may be more suitable than a TURP for your particular circumstances. If you are on anti-coagulation medications, for instance, a laser procedure is a very good choice for reducing a moderate-sized gland. If, however, your prostate is larger than 150 g, consider the holmium laser enucleation or a retropubic prostatectomy.

In the lifetime of an adult male there is more than a fifty percent chance of developing symptoms from an enlarging prostate. All the more reason then for you to view this problem as you would a receding hairline, or the need for bifocals. Never for one moment should you deny yourself a chance to live a full and enjoyable life. You may not be able to ejaculate as you did when you were younger, for instance, but your orgasms will be just as satisfying. More important, you will be able to urinate so much better.

Aspects of care following prostate surgery are fairly uniform, although details may vary from hospital to hospital. At the Royal Victoria Hospital, a man comes in for routine pre-operative assessments about two weeks before his operation. The resident doctor goes over the patient's medical history, examines him fully, and arranges for an electrocardiogram as well as urine and blood tests, of which the PSA is only one. The resident will also consider a cross-match if there is a possibility that a patient may need a blood transfusion.

The anaesthesiologist then arrives to discuss whether a patient should have a regional or a general anaesthetic. Whatever the choice, the patient will be told to clean out his bowels with a powerful laxative the evening before surgery. Usually, he is admitted to hospital the day of his operation having had nothing to eat or drink after midnight.

At the Royal Vic, retropubic prostatectomies are carried out in a regular operating theatre, TURPs and laser prostatectomies in a room designed especially for them. This is because each of these operations requires as much as twelve litres of irrigating fluid to flush out clotting blood and tissue, and regular operating rooms have not been designed with floor-drainage systems that can carry this waste away.

After surgery, whatever the procedure, the patient will have a catheter installed. Pain control medications are routinely prescribed, and blood tests are carried out again to check the degree of blood loss and levels of the natural blood ingredients.

A patient is commonly discharged from hospital after an overnight stay with the catheter removed and with comfortable urinations. On rare occasions, the patient fails his voiding trial and must have the catheter reinserted. He may then be discharged wearing a catheter and be brought back a week later for another voiding trial, which is usually successful. Patients who have had a holmium laser removal of the enlarged prostate usually have a voiding trial the next day, just like the standard TURP patient, and do just as well even if the gland was over 100 g. Patients who have undergone a retropubic prostatectomy may require a longer hospitalization, although discharge with a catheter is possible after 48-72 hours.

With minor variations, this is what to expect should you have surgery for prostate enlargement. You can avoid post-operative complications by breathing deeply even if it hurts, by wriggling your toes, and by getting out of bed as often as you can to prevent inflammation of the leg veins (phlebitis), as well as by taking no

65

more painkillers than is absolutely necessary because these tend to make breathing more shallow, which invites pneumonia and causes constipation.

Post-surgery constipation can be a menacing problem, and it is best alleviated by such bowel softeners as Colace (docusate), and by drinking plenty of water that will also flush out the bladder and release blood clots.

Never be alarmed if suddenly your urine looks bloody again. Sudden appearance of a bloody urine after days of clear urine can occur any time within six weeks after prostate surgery. Patients are thus advised not to travel to remote areas for six weeks.

If you are cheerful, optimistic, and flexible you will get better care and come out ahead.

8

PROSTATITIS:
Bacterial

Of the three major maladies that afflict the prostate, the one most frequently misdiagnosed – and mismanaged – is prostatitis, which can either be infectious or non-infectious, acute or chronic. It's worth mentioning here that ten percent of all office visits to urologists, and one percent of all visits to family doctors, are due to various forms of prostatitis. One quarter of all visits to urologists by men between the age of twenty-five and fifty are for "prostatitis."

This whole area of prostate health, however, is not as clear as it could be, not only among general practitioners but all too frequently among urologists as well. The result is that prostatitis caused by bacteria (an infection) is often confused with a form of prostatitis – which can be just as debilitating – that is likely to be the result of a non-bacterial inflammation.

The problem is complicated further when we consider that non-bacterial prostatitis may have started as a bacterial disease, and that even though the infection may have been eliminated, it remains as an inflammation and continues to cause the patient a lot of pain and distress. Indeed, one problem often mimics the other, and the patient may have both forms of prostatitis simultaneously.

Broadly speaking, prostatitis simply means inflammation of the prostate, just as tonsillitis is inflammation of the tonsils, tendonitis is inflammation of the tendon, or pharyngitis is inflammation of the pharynx.

ACUTE BACTERIAL PROSTATITIS

Acute prostatitis is caused by a massive invasion of bowel bacteria into the prostate gland, a condition quite easily diagnosed because the bacteria are isolated in either blood, urine, or semen, or in all three. Thus, the urologist can examine any one of these components to reach a positive diagnosis. This is usually done by sending a blood or urine sample to a laboratory for culture.

Many years ago, a Danish bacteriologist by the name of Hans Christian Joachim Gram (1853-1938) discovered that all bacteria could be identified by staining them with a dye that turns them either red or blue. Since then, doctors have used this system, and the term "Gram-positive" has come to denote one strain of bacterium while "Gram-negative" defines another. It is the Gram-negative bacteria – those that stain blue with this method – that are the usual cause of bacterial prostatitis.

Other organisms, such as viruses or the tubercle bacilli (the bacteria that cause tuberculosis), or those associated with sexually transmitted organisms like chlamydia and gonorrhoea, do not usually cause prostatitis, although tuberculous prostatitis and chlamydial prostatitis have, on very rare occasions, been described.

How the bowel bacteria actually enter the prostate gland – whether from the bloodstream, via the lymph system, through the urethra, by travelling down the urinary tract from the kidney or the bladder, or by direct extension through the bowel wall – has not been positively ascertained.

Can bacteria from a bad tooth enter the bloodstream and settle in the prostate? Can an infected toenail resulting in a huge and swollen lymph node in the groin create the route for the bacteria? Can diverticulitis, an infection within a blow-out in the intestine, lead to a direct invasion of bacteria to the prostate from the bowel?

The route of prostate infection may not be known, but the clinical manifestations of such a bacterial assault are clear. The patient suddenly falls sick with a high temperature and chills. He may need to urinate very frequently, experience painful urination, or be unable to postpone urination. In some cases, he may not be able to urinate at all.

How is acute bacterial prostatitis diagnosed? When I place my gloved finger in the rectum of a patient I suspect of suffering from this, my suspicions are confirmed when I encounter a hot and spongy prostate gland. I must remember not to carry out a vigorous rectal examination, though, because by inadvertently massaging the gland I might force a large amount of bacteria into the bloodstream and cause more serious problems that are immediately demonstrated by a high fever (septicaemia) that can lead to a collapse of the cardiovascular system. This, the direct result of bacterial products called endotoxins in the bloodstream, used to have a twenty-five percent fatality rate. It is less ominous today because infectious disease specialists have learned to treat the condition more vigorously.

Nevertheless, it is a condition not unlike the bacterial invasion popularly known as "flesh-eating disease." Treatment must be both prompt and very aggressive.

Even without a rectal examination and the accidental massaging of the prostate, a blood culture is always positive because a small amount of bacteria has invariably found its way into the bloodstream. It is always discovered in a urine culture, too. The most likely delinquent organisms are E.coli, followed, in order of frequency of occurrence, by proteus, klebsiella, enterobacter, pseudomonas, and serratia.

Before a patient's culture results come back to my attention, I have already started his treatment for prostatitis with intravenous antibiotics. How can I possibly prescribe antibiotics without the benefit of laboratory results? The answer is quite simple. The condition is usually serious enough to warrant a judgment call – and a quick one. I prescribe antibiotics based on my experience of having treated similar cases in the past. The point is that some kind of treatment must begin immediately, or there may be a high price to pay.

Almost without exception, I am happy to say, my choice of medications turns out to be correct. Gentamicin (between 1 g and 2 g daily intravenously) and ampicillin (2 g four times daily) are the usual first-line drugs for acute bacterial prostatitis. They are administered together.

When these cannot be used because of an allergy, perhaps, or when the patient's kidneys are functioning poorly, quinoline antibiotics like Cipro (200 mg to 400 mg every twelve hours intravenously) are in order. Being kidney-toxic, Gentamicin should not be used.

Sometimes I might prescribe a drug like Kefzol (cefazolin) at the rate of 1 g intravenously every eight hours. The clinical response is almost always prompt and dramatic, and when the patient is well enough, he is switched to oral antibiotics for a few extra weeks. Almost all patients are cured by these medications.

If a patient does not respond promptly to antibiotics and continues to have a spiking temperature (normal in the morning and rising to 103-104 degrees Fahrenheit, or 39 degrees centrigrade, in the afternoon), I worry about an abscess in the prostate.

As is the case of an abscess anywhere else in the body, a prostate abscess must be drained. For the prostate this is best accomplished through the urethra in a procedure not unlike the TURP. The procedure will require an anaesthetic and a few excursions with a resectoscope. We know the abscess is draining when we see pus oozing from the incised prostate.

The urgent necessity of this procedure is best illustrated by recalling another of my patients, a forty-seven-year-old auto mechanic who came to the emergency room in dire distress. He was flushed with fever, had a racing heartbeat, and could barely pass water. The attending physician diagnosed an acute urinary tract infection, and, after routine urine and blood cultures had been rushed off to the laboratory, the patient was immediately given antibiotics.

After he had been admitted to a medical ward for observation, the man seemed to improve. Later, however, he developed urinary retention, and a urology resident was called in to install an indwelling Foley catheter. At this point, after detecting a red-hot prostate on rectal examination, the resident diagnosed acute prostatitis.

Over the next ten days, the patient's afternoon temperature spikes of dangerously high fevers did not abate. A prostatic abscess was discovered by a CT scan, and a resectoscopic drainage of the prostate was carried out. The results were dramatic. As soon as pus oozed from his incised prostate, the patient's high temperature disappeared. From then on, his recovery was swift and smooth.

I have drained a prostatic abscess a number of times in my career, but not all prostate abscesses are close to the urinary passage. Sometimes the abscess is on the outer aspect of the prostate, and the drainage is best performed through the skin.

How do we tell whether the abscess is in the inner or outer aspect of the prostate gland? Clinically, the internal examination called a cystoscopy will reveal a red bulging lump distorting the normal passage within the prostate. More often, a trans-rectal ultrasound examination of the prostate will reveal the abscess, and the person doing the examination, a urologist or a radiologist, will drain the abscess with a needle through the skin under ultra-sound guidance.

CHRONIC BACTERIAL PROSTATITIS

The chronic form of prostatitis is much more enigmatic. Three clinical types are recognized: chronic bacterial prostatitis, chronic non-bacterial prostatitis, and prostatodynia, which is chronic pain that emanates from the prostatic area, or is merely presumed to do so.

71

I see a number of patients who have been treated with antibiotics regardless of their conditions. Many have come to me for a second or third opinion because the pills have not done them any good. When I ask them if medications were prescribed following urine cultures, they very often tell me they hadn't given urine samples at all. When I want to know if a prostatic massage had been carried out as a diagnostic measure, the answer is again negative. The pills were prescribed, I am left to conclude, on the basis of the patients' stories and their doctors' guesses.

At the same time, I see patients who have been dismissed as whiners who have been ascribed low thresholds for pain and discomfort when, according to my assessment, they do indeed have chronic bacterial prostatitis.

Chronic bacterial prostatitis is the diagnosis made most frequently with inadequate diagnostic criteria, sometimes correctly and other times not. Typically, the patient will be a young to middle-aged man who is sexually active and who has a history of previous urinary tract infections. His complaints will include fatigue and malaise, low back pain, irritation or pain on urination (dysuria), and a much-too-frequent need to urinate both day and night. He will also have an itchy urethra while urinating or not, pain or discomfort when sitting, pain during ejaculation or after it, loss of sexual desire, loss of erection, emotional distress, even depression.

It may surprise you to know that a diagnosis of chronic bacterial prostatitis is quite often made purely on the basis of symptoms that later turn out to be psychological – symptoms based entirely on what a patient says about himself and how he describes his problem. Many of these cases involve men who have a guilty conscience for having committed sexual indiscretions, or who have valid clinical depression.

Suffice it to say, then, that it is impossible to base a treatment for chronic bacterial prostatitis based solely on a patient's complaints, especially if treatment might lead to surgery. One thirty-four-year-old graduate student had this dilemma exactly. His urologist was treating him for erectile dysfunction and, when all treatments proved unsuccessful, suggested installing a penile prosthesis.

Understandably, the patient was in a terrible panic when he came to see me. He was indeed impotent, as I discovered. More to the point, he had other symptoms, but having become absolutely preoccupied with his inability to have an erection, he had minimized these.

The fluid I obtained from this patient by prostatic massage showed that he suffered from classic chronic bacterial prostatitis, and this was the source of his erectile dysfunction. I am happy to report that I was able to eradicate the man's prostatitis with antimicrobial therapy, and his potency returned within a matter of weeks. I can assure you that this man was happier than I was for having cured him.

Recently, urologists have devised a system – yet to be fully accepted by the specialty at large – to try to ascertain if symptom scores, like the IPSS, which helps define the severity of an enlarged prostate, could help differentiate between prostatitis that is real and prostatitis that is purely psychological.

The system isn't perfect, of course, and that is why respectable urologists have, under the pressure of unending work, been known to prescribe drugs for patients who do not have prostatitis at all, only some of its peripheral symptoms. We know, of course, that if a man has blood in his urine, and a combination of other blatant symptoms associated with prostatitis, he certainly has the disease.

What we need to ascertain now, however, is what to do when a man displays only some of the less severe symptoms that might, on close examination, be attributed to something else.

The point is, it is really impossible to make a prostatitis diagnosis on the basis of a man's complaints – that it is painful to sit, that his penis hurts, that his prostate feels tender when he ejaculates – when no examination has been done to ascertain that there are more telling signs and symptoms.

DIAGNOSIS

The classical and time-honoured method for diagnosing chronic bacterial prostatitis is a quantitative urine culture done before and after prostatic massage. Bacterial counts should be ten times higher in the urine specimen obtained after prostatic massage than in a first one or in a mid-stream urine sample.

Although this test was first reported in 1968 by the Americans Dr. Edwin Meares and Dr. Thomas Stamey, and remains the "gold standard," it is seldom done. A Canadian expert, Dr. Curtis Nickel, at Queen's University in Kingston, Ontario, has suggested why: the test is enormously time-consuming, and the monetary reward for establishing the correct diagnosis is disproportionate to the effort involved.

It takes at least half an hour to collect the urine sample, carry out a prostatic massage, and collect a second sample. According to government-run Medicare schemes, the monetary reward for correctly diagnosing chronic bacterial prostatitis is a fraction of the reward for seeing three patients in the same time-frame and making an incorrect diagnosis in all three cases.

Furthermore, patients cannot always void on command after prostatic massage. Thus, most clinicians resort to the examination of the prostatic fluid after massage, looking for the presence of leucocytes (white blood cells) and macrophages that contain fat (oval fat bodies) under the microscope.

When there are fewer than fifteen white blood cells per high-power field at forty times magnification, the test is negative. When there are more than fifteen cells, often in clumps, the test is positive.

The massage should not be done within forty-eight hours after the patient has ejaculated. Prostatic massage within forty-eight hours of ejaculation may show spuriously high readings of leucocytes, or may not yield fluid for examination. Although the presence of leucocytes is not synonymous with the presence of bacteria, it is nonetheless a marker – and better than guesswork.

I once spoke to a gathering of primary care physicians and suggested that microscopy should be mandatory in the absence of sequential urine cultures to diagnose chronic bacterial prostatitis. A doctor in the audience rightly pointed out that microscopes were not part of the paraphernalia in a normal primary care practice. In this case, primary care physicians must not try to diagnose chronic bacterial prostatitis.

I began testing prostatic massage secretion on the leucocyte band of the dipstick and compared it to examination under the microscope at forty times magnification. I can now say that the leucocyte band on the dipstick can be used as a good substitute for microscopy. A dark purple, or a two-plus, reading corresponds to fifteen or more leucocytes per high-power field. If the dipstick contains a nitrite band, it is even possible to distinguish bacterial prostatitis from non-bacterial prostatitis. The nitrite band becomes positive when bacteria are present, not when leucocytes are present on their own.

Once the diagnosis of chronic bacterial prostatitis is established, anti-microbial therapy is begun. I use Floxin (ofloxacin) or, more recently, Levaquin, and the trimethoprim-sulfamethoxazole combination of Septra or Bactrim, alternating the two drugs every two weeks for a minimum treatment of twelve weeks. After that, I often ask patients to take half the dosage – 300 mg of Floxin daily instead of twice a day, or one double strength Septra instead of two, for a month – before halving it further every month, until only half a pill is taken each day for up to a year. When patients relapse, the dosage is raised to the starting dose.

In addition to taking anti-microbial drugs, I advise patients to cut out alcohol, coffee, and spices, ejaculate frequently, and bring heat to the prostatic area by taking hot baths or sitz baths. Most patients respond, but the problem often recurs.

The choice of Floxin and Septra or Bactrim deserves amplification. Floxin is one of the quinoline antibiotics, like Cipro (ciprofloxacin) and Noroxin (norfloxacin). Floxin has been displaced by Levaquin (levfloxin), which is a 500 mg daily pill. Cipro is probably the most widely used quinoline today. It is well tolerated and very effective for most Gram-negative bacterial invasions of the body. Noroxin is well tolerated, too, and remains the best "strong" pill for the routine urinary infection. Cipro and Noroxin, though, do not diffuse into the prostate as well as Levaquin.

Septra was developed in the Burroughs Wellcome laboratories headed by the late Dr. George Hitchings. In my lecture to medical students I often extol Hitchings's genius. Here was a man, outside academia, who had a major impact on the practice of medicine. His team developed Zyloprim (allopurinol), which has forever altered the management of gout and uric acid elevation, and he introduced rejection-fighting Imuran (azathioprine), which launched the possibility of organ transplantation. He then introduced Septra, which was a combination of sulfamethoxazole and trimethoprim.

Here, however, I think he made a multi-billion dollar blunder. There is nothing wrong with this combination drug, but trimethoprim could have been combined with another sulphonamide rather than Hoffmann-La Roche's patent-protected sulfamethoxazole.

If a trimethoprim-sulphadiazine combination had been released first, Burroughs Wellcome would not have had to share the initial profits with Hoffmann-La Roche. The combination would have worked just as well, and the company coffers might have been enhanced by billions of dollars. Clever people do sometimes make colossal miscalculations.

Perhaps there is another side to this story. Maybe the best results in the Burroughs Wellcome laboratories occurred with the combination of trimethoprim and sulfamethoxazole over trimethoprim and sulphadiazine. Rather than release an inferior product, the folks at Burroughs Wellcome favoured science over profit.

I will stick to my story, though. The trimethoprim-sulphadiazine combination constitutes a product that is just as good in terms of bacterial coverage and effectiveness, has no increased side effects, and is a smaller pill that is easy to swallow.

I treat my patients with chronic bacterial prostatitis for twelve weeks on the full dosage of quinolones or sulphonamide-trimethoprim combination, and even for a longer time on reduced dosages, like one half pill every other day. Should there be a relapse, patients return to the full dosage for an indeterminate period.

If prolonged anti-bacterial therapy has any merit at all it must be because indolent bacteria hiding within the prostate are difficult to eradicate. It makes sense, then, to heat the prostate to temperatures that can kill bacteria without causing excessive tissue injury – to about 40 degrees centrigrade.

Such a rationale is behind hyperthermia treatment of the prostate, which we have already talked about. The same machine used to treat enlarged prostates has been tried on patients with prostatitis. In an enlarged prostate, mild heat did not change the urinary flow rate nor the size of the gland, but it nonetheless made patients feel better.

Could they have been treated for chronic bacterial prostatitis instead? Investigators in Israel and Italy have explored the use of hyperthermia to treat prostatitis, and some encouraging results have been reported. So much so that I have sent some of my patients for hyperthermia treatment. The treatment is available in Canada but is not usually covered by Medicare schemes.

Almost all patients report some improvement with hyperthermia treatment, but I do not know if they are merely trying to rationalize the money they have spent to have it, or if the heat may have killed their pain by killing nerve endings. I would like to think that the treatment also killed bacteria.

The terrible consequences of severe bacterial prostatitis is probably best illustrated by another patient — a fifty-eight-year-old family practitioner, no less, who displayed all the symptoms associated with this chronic disease. He had read the first edition of my book *Private Parts* and felt I was describing him when I wrote about "symptoms that may combine to make life seem not worth living."

This physician asked me to take him on as a patient, and I agreed. I persuaded him to try all the different medications available for bacterial prostatitis, as well as hyperthermia, which, as I have explained, is a suspect treatment for prostate enlargement, but which might nonetheless help prostatitis.

When hyperthermia failed, the patient persuaded me to surgically remove as much of the offending prostate tissue as I could, and this I agreed to do in a procedure I likened to a drastic TURP. Alas, this brought only brief and temporary relief.

Finally, the patient and I both agreed on a more drastic solution: the radical removal of his prostate, a procedure usually reserved only for cancer.

Fortunately, the outcome was successful, and the patient has never regretted taking this step. I had warned him that the operation could render him impotent or incontinent or both. Chronic bacterial prostatitis had left him with an infection so deep and painful that he was willing to take the chance.

9

PROSTATITIS:
Non-bacterial

The symptoms of non-bacterial prostatitis are indistinguishable from those of chronic bacterial prostatitis, but there is no infection. In other words, non-bacterial prostatitis is really inflammation of the prostate, and this causes the same kind of irritation as we would expect when bacteria are present.

Were bacteria present originally, but eliminated by antibiotics? Are bacteria present but undetectable, hiding under a bio-film (a thin protein layer like veneer on plywood)? Or were bacteria absent in the first place?

The answers to these questions are not always readily forthcoming. Perhaps some cases of chronic, non-bacterial prostatitis are originally due to bacteria, while others have been caused by a urine backflow into the prostatic ducts, causing an inflammatory reaction not unlike reflux nephropathy.

In reflux nephropathy, which is a disorder that primarily affects pre-school children, urine is regurgitated from the bladder into the kidney tissue, where it initiates an inflammation that can scar down a kidney. Severely damaged, shrunken, almost non-functioning kidneys have been the result of severe cases of childhood reflux nephropathy.

Experiments done by filling the bladder through a catheter with water containing Indian ink show that urine can, under a certain set of circumstances, penetrate the prostatic ducts. This investigative test was carried out some years ago when a handful of patients, each about to undergo a TURP for an enlarged prostate, volunteered to have Indian ink instilled into their bladders via a Foley catheter three days before their operations. Doctors in charge of the study discovered that prostatic ducts in the carved-out prostate tissue contained the ink much more often in those patients with a known history of chronic non-bacterial prostatitis than in those who had no such history. This means that the regurgitation of urine into the prostatic ducts may well be the way in which chronic non-bacterial prostatitis occurs.

Whatever the natural course the disease may have taken – where it began, and how and why – I usually treat my non-bacterial prostatitis patients with the same course of anti-microbial drugs (Septra or Levaquin, for example) that I would use if the bacteria were present. I do this on the simple presumption that the problem might have a bacterial component. If patients respond to these drugs – and many do – I continue the treatment as if their problems were bacterial, even thought they might be otherwise.

If there is no response at all, I stop this treatment and substitute the antibiotics with non-steroidal anti-inflammatory drugs. These include either Indocid (indomethacin) or Naprosyn (naproxen), or the Cox-2 inhibitors like Celebrex (celecoxib). Will medications that treat nerve pains associated with diabetes or shingles, like Lyrica (pregabalind) find a role to play for this condition? It remains to be seen. I do add a muscle relaxant such as Valium (diazepam) at times. I may also try Prosta (quercetin), a bioflavonoid dietary supplement that was found effective in a scientific study. The number of patients who have responded to anti-inflammatory drugs are few and far between, I have to admit.

When or if pain is a major factor, I add a night-time dosage of 10 mg of Elavil (amytriptylline), building up to a dosage of 25 mg, and occasionally 75 mg. Patients are not always rendered pain free with this, but many say they are helped by it when nothing else has worked. Sometimes a patient needs to be referred to a pain clinic or a psychologist, even a psychiatrist, because I feel he is harbouring an underlying problem that I, as a urologist, am just not equipped to deal with. I have had much more success with amytriptylline than with Lyrica (pregabaalind), a drug that controls nerve source pain.

Consider the man who did the rounds of Montreal dentists asking them to remove his teeth because, he said, they ached incessantly. Eventually, after several extractions, he met a dentist who told him that his problem was in his head and not his mouth. He needed a psychiatrist because his dental pain was psychosomatic.

Such was the case of a fifty-two-year-old man who, when referred to me by his family doctor, was miserable with low back pain. He also had pain in his prostate area, pain in his upper thighs, pain on urination, pain on ejaculation, pain in his groin, pain in his lower abdomen, pain everywhere. The only positive finding was the presence of numerous leucocytes in fluid I obtained after performing a prostatic massage.

Antibiotics did not help him, which suggested that there was no infection. Anti-inflammatory drugs, such as Naprosyn and Indocid, were just as ineffective, as were painkillers like Codeine and Percocet. Some relief, however, was obtained by combining Valium, Elavil, and the anti-depressant Prozac (fluoxetine), but the patient's symptoms were still far from being controlled.

At present, he is coping with his discomfort, though he has virtually no sex life and must often be absent from work. In the future, he knows he may well need to seek help not only from a specialist in pain control, but from a psychiatrist as well. I believe that his discomfort, severe as it is, is largely stress-related.

PROSTATODYNIA

Although the pain associated with prostatodynia is in the area of the prostate, it has nothing to do with the gland itself. Urine cultures done before and after prostate massage are always bacteria-free, and leucocytes are invariably absent from prostatic secretion. The problem is presumed to originate from disorders of the muscles in the pelvic floor. Geographically, then, it appears to be the domain of the urologist when, in fact, it is really not urological at all.

Nonetheless, I treat it. A strong non-steroidal anti-inflammatory drug, like Toradol (ketorolac tromethamine), may help some patients, and I often try this medication before all others.

If the patient's urine flow is poor, I prescribe an alpha-blocker like Flomax, Xytral, Rapaflo, Cardura, or Hytrin. Treatment for prostatodynia with Elmiron (pentosan polysulfate), a drug for a bladder condition known as interstitial cystitis, has helped a few patients.

Interstitial cystitis is a predominantly female ailment with many unknowns. No one knows, for example, what causes it, how best to diagnose it, nor even the most reliable way to treat it. Urologists are also bemused as to why it affects women ninety percent of the time.

What we *do* know, however, is that this aggravating condition is linked to the absence of a fine, protective layer of protein called glycos-amino-glycan (GAG) which lines the inner surface of the bladder to prevent urine from seeping into the bladder walls. In a healthy adult, that layer is there. Just as the protective coating of Teflon prevents food from sticking to a frying pan, the GAG makes the surface of the bladder less sticky to bacteria and blocks urine from seeping into the lining first, then underlying layers of muscle later.

In interstitial cystitis, much of this GAG is lost, and urine is able to seep into bladder muscles, creating a nasty inflammation. This, in turn, causes severe pain, particularly as the bladder fills up. It lessens as the bladder is emptied, but starts up again as the cycle is repeated.

Because the severe pain of this condition mimics that of non-bacterial prostatitis, or prostatodynia, Elmiron is being explored as a possibly effective medication. We now have data to show that Elmiron is effective, but only in a minority of cases.

10

PROSTATITIS:
The Last Word

The more I think about it, the more I realize that I wouldn't wish prostatitis – acute or chronic, bacterial, or non-bacterial – on anyone. It is all too often a diabolical disorder, debilitating and depressing, that has a man agonizing for days on end until his medications finally kick in. Sometimes, medications don't kick in at all, and the patient is left wondering whether he'll ever live without pain or urinate and ejaculate without pain again.

In truth, urologists don't much like treating this condition at all because good, lasting results take a lot of time, if they occur at all. They would much rather deal with a tumour or a kidney stone because conditions such as these enable them to see the results of their work relatively quickly.

Should you be unfortunate enough to become afflicted with prostatitis, there are a number of safeguards you should remember. First, you should insist upon all the necessary diagnostic measures we have been discussing. Anti-microbial therapy should err on the side of over-treatment rather than under-treatment. Anti-inflammatory medications, muscle relaxants, painkillers and other drugs can only be assessed on a trial-and-error basis.

There is no controversy about how to diagnose and treat bacterial prostatitis either, if it is acute or chronic. Non-bacterial prostatitis and prostatodynia are, of course, far different matters. Because there are no specific diagnostic criteria for these – nor established treatments, for that matter – they are mysterious entities indeed, and, consequently, they lend themselves to all manner of witchcraft and quackery.

Much of this morass of deception, intentional or otherwise, is perpetrated most widely on the Internet. Here, information is disseminated at will without its being peer-reviewed or subjected to any kind of editorial scrutiny. A person need only be able to type, after all, to have access to the Internet, either to gather information, or to post it there.

Of course, there is nothing at all wrong with a person lamenting his misfortunes on the Internet. Patients can, almost anonymously, spill out their hearts on the most private of matters. They may describe their battles with what they may think is prostatitis, for instance, and how every expert urologist has failed them.

Conversely, they often describe "successful" experiences with alternative medicines and their trials with different herbs and nutritional supplements, some of which have no medical value whatsoever. Indeed, people are able to speak at will on the Internet, on anything.

There is, however, something inherently evil when unqualified people speak of predictable cures for things that may be incurable, and even more so when they promote costly treatments without having submitted their results for scientific evaluation.

It amazes me how the new information age has transformed the way in which we look at disease. In the "good old days," the physician was king, and everyone deferred to his (or her) wisdom and experience. Today, many patients walk into a doctor's office with a wealth of "information" garnered from websites, from good friends "whose father had exactly what I have," and from quacks and charlatans who advertise on websites and even in print media. Today's physician has to be aware of all this when a patient enters the office, as a goodly amount of time may have to be set aside to debunk myths before the patient will be willing to try a "gold standard" treatment, which differs from the latest fad.

I have seen instances where men have talked glowingly on the Internet about the so-called cures claimed by an "expert" in the Philippines who diligently carries out repeated prostatic massages on his long-suffering patients with miraculous results! This doctor's claims of cures seem incredible to me, yet numerous patients make the long trek to the Philippines especially to consult him, and many offer testimonials to his "skills."

I do not think that this doctor is necessarily an outright fraud, because I suspect there may be substantial benefits in the frequent, and repeated, prostate massages he advocates. There is something wrong, however, with this whole scenario because diseases such as chronic non-bacterial prostatitis almost always take many sessions to control, but are never really cured. In this they are like a smoker's chronic bronchitis, which will almost always recur from time to time. Besides, this doctor's urological credentials could be better. Thankfully, more traditional urological treatments for prostatitis prevail. I believe, however, that those doctors who administer them should become more creative in their approach to this all-too-prevalent ailment.

Why is this internal gland we know as the prostate so sensitive to pain? Why does it seem to attract bacteria so easily? Why does it swell much more frequently than other glands?

Doctors who have chosen to specialize in this field might ask themselves such questions so as to better understand the entire scope of prostate disorders.

They might also ask: why are structures that are attached to the prostate, like the seminal vesicles (one of organs that produces some of the ejaculate fluid), or the vas deferens (tubes that transport sperm from the testicles to the prostate), almost without sensation or disease when the gland itself is so susceptible to pain and inflammation?

To best illustrate this, I should mention my technique for performing a vasectomy. Although I freeze the skin of the scrotum, I am able to pluck out the vas just beneath, clamp it, cut it, then cauterize it — all with no extra anaesthetic. Also, I have seen men with large cysts on their seminal vesicles, or impressive distensions of them, who have experienced no pain at all because, like the vas, the seminal vesicles have few nerve endings, while the prostate has many.

When we further consider prostate disease, we might look to other organs for help — the lungs, for instance. Indeed, in some ways, the lungs and the prostate are similar. Lungs are subject to cancer, degenerative enlargement (emphysema), and infection (pneumonia), just as the prostate can develop cancer, enlargement, or prostatitis. But, lungs are also subject to asthma, bronchiectasis, pleurisy, so there may be prostatic equivalents that are, at present, all lumped together under the umbrella term we know only as prostatitis.

This should cause us urologists to think that we might perhaps expand our thinking on this topic — that there could be more than merely three conditions that can adversely affect the prostate .

The presence of certain chemicals may help us do this. For instance, one of the perplexing facts of human anatomy is that there is more zinc residing in the prostate than anywhere else in the body. No one seems to know why this is, or if the quantity of zinc is a factor in disease development. This may also be true of other trace metals, including cadmium and copper.

We know, too, that the protein made by prostate cells — the all-important PSA — makes the gelatinous ejaculate liquid, but again, we cannot ascertain how important this is to fertility. We have also discovered that the seminal vesicles mysteriously manufacture a fruit-sugar substance called fructose and that a sperm taken from the testicle or epididymis before contact with the prostate or seminal vesicle can create a normal baby. But the precise details of these phenomena also remain a mystery.

What then is the meaning of these findings within the prostate and the attached seminal vesicles? It is important that we learn the answers to these questions so we can find out if, perhaps, there is a disease that is related to zinc disturbances, which can affect the prostate, or if there is a muscle disorder, like asthma, that can specifically attack prostate muscle cells. In this case, prostatic duct disorders, like a bronchiectasis, might be more significant than we think.

There are other relevant questions. Could frequent, almost daily, prostatic massages make a difference to prostate health, and should a more vigorous massage under an anaesthetic become a serious consideration for long-term treatment? Can chemical cautery, with alcohol or phenol, destroy nerve endings and relieve symptoms? Can the direct infusion of drugs into the prostate, with ultrasound guidance, play a role in the future treatment of enlargement and prostatitis, even cancer?

With answers to these questions we urologists might be able to further refine our craft and determine the entire spectrum of what can ail a once-healthy prostate gland, and, more important, what can heal it.

Finally, prostatitis does not need the exclusive attention of a urologist – only when it is acute and requires surgical drainage, which must be done in hospital under the supervision of a urology team. Chronic prostatitis, on the other hand, merely requires an empathetic family physician who is willing and able to carry out simple diagnostic measures, provide pragmatic support, and demonstrate the way to recovery of a complex disease.

On this note, there is no need for despair. Always remember that if ever you are diagnosed with severe prostatitis, you should ensure that any treatment you have been given, which may at first appear ineffective, is afforded a proper chance to succeed. Don't expect overnight miracles.

11

PROSTATE CANCER:
Who Will Get It and Why?

One of the most frightening diseases in our world is cancer. Despite the fact that wonderful progress has been made in many fields of medicine, cancer remains an enigma. It is a condition that changes even as we struggle to cope with it in its present incarnation. The prostate is only one of many organs that can be targeted by this disease, and when it strikes, it is the combination of speedy diagnosis and prompt and appropriate treatment that can make the difference between a return to full health and a difficult path to more serious consequences.

Unless medical science advances, and diets and lifestyles change, fourteen percent of all baby boys born each year in the early part of the twenty-first century will develop prostate cancer, the second most common cancer in all males, and one that is outnumbered only by skin cancer. Twenty-five percent of these same males will actually die from the disease. As a killing cancer, prostate cancer is second only to lung cancer.

In the United States, of just under 200,000 men who are newly diagnosed with the disease each year, approximately 40,000 will succumb to it. And, according to the Canadian Cancer Society, every year, more than 16,000 Canadian men will be told they have prostate cancer, and it will kill about 4,000 of them.

All this, of course, is the bad news. The good news is that thanks to the strides science has been able to make over the past few decades, such a death rate need not occur at all. One of the main problems of prostate cancer is that it more often masquerades as either an enlarged prostate or a simple case of prostatitis. In its infancy, it will display no symptoms at all. Nonetheless, early diagnosis and the correct medical or surgical treatment almost always translate into a complete cure.

All this must be considered in another light. Those men who are killed by prostate cancer will be victims of what is known as "the tiger" – a lethal, fast-moving form of the disease, while others will suffer the considerably slower-growing form known as "the pussy cat." Life with a slower-growing prostate cancer is almost always sustained for many years, if not decades, with virtually no ill effects other than the psychological impact of having the disease.

Broadly speaking, prostate cancer can be either a "pussy-cat" that may never prove fatal, or a "tiger" which, without treatment, certainly will. It is heartening to remember, however, that even those men who have the severest form of this dreaded disease – especially those in their seventies and beyond – usually die *with* it rather than *from* it.

Is prostate cancer an epidemic?

In medicine, we tend to apply the term "epidemic" only to a disease that is widespread and that is passed from one person to another, like the common cold or an influenza virus. But the word may also be used to define something that is extremely prevalent. So, given the numbers, prostate cancer may indeed qualify as an epidemic. A one-in-seven chance of contracting a form of cancer that can be fatal if left untreated is a startling and frightening statistic that raises the issue of what is an epidemic more pungently than ever.

The next point we must consider is this: if prostate cancer *is* an epidemic, how should public health officials – doctors, nurses, administrators, and politicians, to name just a few – deal with it? Urologists, who are the primary health care providers for a disease that is so obviously pegged to the growing number of greying Baby Boomers as they amble through the years – could sure use the help.

The management of any widely distributed health problem involves five levels of medical activity: health promotion, specific prevention, early diagnosis and treatment, disease limitation, and rehabilitation. Some of these are concurrent and others sequential, and I will discuss them all in due course. First, though, let me talk about all the preventative measures I feel comfortable in touting, the ongoing issue of genetic predisposition to prostate cancer, and the possibility that the disease may finally be licked, in the not-too-distant future, by genetic manipulation that may entail a simple inoculation.

THE CHEMISTRY OF PROSTATE CANCER

The biochemical changes in a man's body that promote the development of prostate cancer are just beginning to be understood. This is a complex topic and one that medical scientists can now explain, though not in its entirety.

The prostate gland develops under the influence of the natural male hormone testosterone, which is manufactured in the testicles and which is ever-present in the adult male. It is this, after all, that not only promotes sexual appetite, but the capacity to satisfy it, too.

Ironically, with the good comes the bad. Testosterone increases the propensity for prostate cancer, too, as we know from the fate of those eunuchs who were castrated before puberty. Those young men developed prostate glands all right, but, without the presence of testosterone, they did not develop either prostate cancer or enlargement.

Testosterone in the blood circulation is largely fixed to a protein called sex hormone-binding globulin (SHBG), and this testosterone is unavailable for use. A small amount, roughly 1-4%, that floats freely and is not fixed or bound to the protein called free testosterone makes its way into the nucleus of the prostate cells. (Some of the free testosterone is loosely bound to albumin and is called bio-available testosterone because it is usable. When a urologist wants to know if the lack of a sex drive, or libido, is due to lack of testosterone, he measures the bio-available testosterone between 9 and 11 in the morning, with normal results expected to be higher than 3.5 nanograms/mL.)

Cancer starts with the transformation of a normal glandular cell into a malignant cell. Theoretically, this change can be seen under the microscope within the nucleus of the cell. I say, theoretically, because the very first change in the very first cell cannot be seen. It would be like finding the needle in a haystack.

Actually, cancer is considered to be multifocal in origin. It is not just one cell but a number of cells that become cancerous, and each cell multiplies repeatedly. By the time a microscope can detect the cancer, there are thousands, hundreds of thousands, probably millions of cells involved. The nucleus of the cancer cell will be larger, and there will be a prominent nucleolus, a structure within the nucleus that becomes more readily apparent.

Now, there will be variations in cell sizes, particularly variation in nuclear sizes, with more than the normal numbers of chromosomes. This is called ploidy analysis, diploid signifying a relatively benign nature, and aneuploid an aggressive cancer. By the time cancer is detectable as a hard spot within the gland, there will usually be several satellite lesions there, too.

It is not clear when malignant cells leave the gland and start lesions in other areas of the body. It appears that in some men the disease will occupy almost the entire gland before it spreads beyond the prostate. In other men, the disease will invade adjacent tissue, like the seminal vesicles, bladder neck, or urethra before it spreads beyond the prostate to the lymph nodes and bone. Some men will have widespread disease, usually in bones, at a time when the disease within the prostate is minuscule.

Thus, rendering proper and accurate advice to patients is not always possible but, as a rule, a person with a low Gleason grade cancer (Gleason 6 or less), associated with a lower PSA count (< 10), with fewer biopsy needles (< 50%) showing cancer with less of the cylinder involved (< 10%), has better odds of outliving this disease than someone at the other extreme in all these parameters.

Also, in the gland, there dwell two cancer-fighting genes. One is called p-53, the other retinoblastoma suppressor. When these genes are damaged, are in short supply, or are totally absent, as is sometimes the case, cancer is promoted by default because there is nothing strong enough to fight it by allowing such cancer-promoting genes as ras proto-oncogene, and another known as c-erb B2, to thrive.

Generally speaking, prostate cancer occurs with the activation of one set of genes and the loss of another that has the power to deter a tumour from ever taking root. The cancer spreads with the loss of a cell-adhesion molecule called E-cadherin and the release of products that promote new blood vessels (angiogenesis). The result of this is that new blood vessels nurture the cancer – and promote its growth.

We are now so certain of this that medical scientists believe that prostate cancer may be controlled by the development of medications that can block the very thing on which tumours may feed, not to mention spread.

HEALTH PROMOTION AND PROSTATE CANCER

Can good health habits, a healthy diet, exercise, freedom from anxiety and malnutrition, an optimistic outlook, lots of laughter, family support, religious faith, community spirit, clean living, vitamins, herbal preparations, and products from "alternative medicine" lower the risks of developing prostate cancer?

There are no trials that have tested any of these factors. Nor can we expect these studies to be carried out because it is generally accepted that they would be far too time-consuming for the amount of information they would unearth. Testimonials, meanwhile, are far from scientific, only ever offering anecdotal evidence.

Trials of the use of food additives and herbal preparations do not come under the jurisdiction, nor even the scrutiny, of such government agencies as the Food and Drug Administration in the United States or the Health Protection Branch in Canada. This means that a maverick business person can freely extract the juice of a turnip, let's say, and market it as a product that claims – fraudulently – to help a man with prostate cancer, and the government can do little about it.

Similarly, cold therapy (cryo-therapy) and heat therapy (thermo-therapy) is not controlled by governmental agencies, either. Ice and fire, after all, have been around for centuries, just like food and food additives. Thus, the public has to make a judgment call. It must decide whether it is for or against these often-useless products and procedures, assessing not only testimonials of well-meaning citizens, but also what may be thinly disguised promotions by entrepreneurial, sometimes unscrupulous, business people who do not have the public's well-being at heart.

At the same time, scientific claims by the professionals are notoriously suspect. A headline that announces a finding often befits a tabloid more than a scientific journal. In January 1999, for example, *The Canadian Medical Association Journal* reported a fifty-nine percent increase in the incidence of testicular cancer between 1964 and 1996. Investigative journalists hounded urologists for a likely explanation. After all, such an increase did seem alarming and was certainly newsworthy.

In truth, however, the incidence had changed from a mere four in 100,000 males to a little more than six in 100,000. This was a sixty percent increase all right, but do two additional cases per 100,000 really represent a rise that is either catastrophic or cause for alarm? I think not.

94

Similarly, a prominent Harvard epidemiologist reported a sixty-percent increased risk of prostate cancer following vasectomies. A sixty-percent increased risk was actually a four percent difference in two populations – those with vasectomies and those without.

Repeated studies at other centres failed to confirm these findings. It was like proving that there were more complications with vasectomies done on Tuesdays than there were with those accomplished on Wednesdays. As Mark Twain so astutely observed many years ago, "There are lies, damn lies, and statistics." Indeed, scientists and physicians are just as guilty of muddying the waters as are product promoters.

As I have expressed my concerns about health promoting products, let me now state my own prejudices.

I believe that the threat of a disease like cancer – prostate cancer included – forever lingers in the mind of the adult male, and that this is increased by both a genetic predisposition to the disease and a weakened immune system. For now, we cannot control the genetic elements of contracting cancer. A weakened immune system, however, is different. This is very definitely a problem we can do something about.

In recent years, two interesting revelations have emerged. First, the immune system is affected by a person's emotional state. Thus a happy and optimistic person will have an immune system working for him – fighting for him – while an unhappy, pessimistic man will not have this protection at all. In this respect, the writer Norman Cousins was right. A joke a day may well keep cancer away.

Second, cancer is more likely to start in a body that is teeming with what are known as "free radicals," a hypothesis first put forward by an American scientist named Dr. Denham Harman. According to high school chemistry, a "free radical" occurs when a molecule has an unpaired electron on its outer orbit. In medical terms it is formed when oxygen carried by the haemoglobin in the red blood cells breaks down sugar in other cells to produce energy; in the process, oxygen acquires an extra electron, an unstable state that can be stabilized by the oxidation of fat, protein, or DNA. This oxidation of fat can cause cholesterol deposits on arteries, while the oxidation of DNA can promote cancer.

Free radicals, then, cause random damage to protein, enzymes, large molecules, and DNA – an attractive hypothesis that jibes with common sense and allows us to do something about it. It is akin to rust on a car body that can be delayed or prevented by rustproofing. That is to say, an extra intake of anti-oxidants can neutralize the damage that the free radicals cause in the human body by curtailing oxidation.

Anti-oxidants are readily available, perhaps most commonly as vitamin C, vitamin E, and beta-carotene. Other sources made familiar to the public include ceruloplasmin, cysteine, glutathione, superoxide dimutase, transferrin, and D-penicillamine. Selenium has an indirect role; a deficiency of selenium affects the action of glutathione.

It makes sense, then, to adopt a lifestyle that would make a person happier and more optimistic. Exercises and diet help maintain a slim and trim body and contribute to a better bodily image and an improved sense of well-being and, possibly, a healthier immune system into the bargain.

An ample intake of vitamin C and vitamin E and maybe extra glutathione (available, for example, as a milk whey product called Immunocal), or powerful anti-oxidants like Pygnogenol can't hurt. Supplemental selenium also makes sense as a cancer-fighting agent, and this is available without a prescription.

SPECIFIC PREVENTION

Wouldn't it be wonderful if we could prevent prostate cancer specifically the way we can prevent polio, measles, diphtheria, or whooping cough: with a vaccine? Why can we not? Why can we not make a vaccine from cancer cells, inoculate all men in their forties, and thereby prevent all prostate tumours?

There are two simple reasons why we can't. First, cancers are as individually specific as the people they attack. Each one is like a fingerprint, possessing its own characteristics that cannot be emulated or duplicated in another person. If, for instance, we could make one person's immune system react to the foreignness of his cancer, it would not follow that we could transfer this response to a second person's cancer, even if both tumours involved dwelled in the prostate.

Second, cancer cells, though foreign, do not normally provoke an immune reaction as they grow and spread throughout the body. It is curious to me that cancer generally spreads first to the nearest lymph node, which, as in the case of a bacterial infection should, ideally, be the first garrison of defence.

To put this another way, I am asking myself why cancer runs wild in the lymph nodes when an ordinary infection is not only contained there, but is subsequently eliminated there – by a lymph node's disease-fighting properties. The lymph nodes do not fight, nor ward off, cancer cells as they do bacterial invasions. Indeed, cancer cells appear to thrive within them. Until we learn why this happens, a cure for advanced forms of cancer may be a long way off.

Meanwhile, the spread of all cancers really amounts to a breakdown in the established bodily defence mechanism. Forty years ago, scientists wondered if spread (metastatic) cancer in the lymph node could give rise to other cancers (metastases), or whether the metastases always had their origins in primary tumours. In a simple and elegant experiment, an investigator successfully transplanted cancer cells from lymph nodes in laboratory rats into those of other rats of the same genetic strain, proving that metastatic lesions can be the source of cancer in other sites.

It is a fact that cancer cells can be made to mount an immune response by being processed by particular cells in the body. These processing cells, or dendritic cells, reside just under the skin as well as within the blood as macrophages. They have been extracted, grown in sterilized bottles outside the body, exposed to irradiated (killed) prostate cancer cells, and then sent back into a patient suffering from the same cancer by a series of injections. An immune reaction against the cancer has been demonstrated, and it has been curtailed or killed. There is justified hope this kind of approach, called experimental immunotherapy, which has been used to combat prostate cancer, will soon make a difference in the development of a vaccine.

The recently approved Dendreon product, called Provenge (sipuleucel-T) shows early promise, but the treatment is extraordinarily expensive, costing about $100,000 per patient.

Exactly how Dendreon made its product remains a proprietory secret. Rather than killed cancer cells, the company cleverly exposed the dendritic cells to acid phosphatase, an enzyme specific to prostate cancer, grew the biologic product in vats outside the body, and injected it back into the patient. It got FDA approval after studies showed that, in advanced disease, life was prolonged by several months.

GENETIC PREDISPOSITION

A genetic predisposition to prostate cancer is present in certain unfortunate families. Prostate cancer in a father makes his son twice as likely to develop the disease, often at a younger age. Prostate cancer in a father and two paternal uncles increases the risk to a son five times, as does the presence of prostate cancer in three successive generations – great-grandfather, grandfather, and father.

The presence of cancer in two brothers under the age of fifty-five also raises the risk for the third brother, by five times. Furthermore, a recent report from France suggested that prostate cancer in a father made his daughters more likely to develop breast cancer.

What would be the risk of prostate cancer if a father and a maternal grandfather both had it?

I don't know the answer to that. What I *do* know is that these familial cancers have been related to a gene alteration on a specific chromosome that is autosomal. That is to say, one that is not a sex chromosome.

Actually, it's a bit more complicated than that, even. There are a number of genes called oncogenes, which promote cancer. There are also suppressor genes that inhibit cancers. The interaction of these – the promoters and the suppressors – within an environment that can be influenced by diet and lifestyle results in a situation that promotes the onset of cancer, or, conversely, the curtailment of it.

RACE, DIET, AND LIFESTYLE

Apart from familial predisposition, race and lifestyle are also contributing factors in the contraction of cancer. Studies show that African-American men are twenty percent more likely to develop prostate cancer than are white Americans, and at a younger age, too. Japanese men, on the other hand, are less likely to develop prostate cancer, but, as is the case with enlarged prostate, after they have lived in North America for more than twenty years their risk becomes as high as that of white Americans.

By way of further elaboration, the risk of a Japanese man developing prostate cancer while living in the industrial city of Osaka is six per 100,000, whereas the risk for an immigrant to San Francisco is sixteen per 100,000. Therefore, factors other than genes – diet, environment, and lifestyle – are thought to play a role.

Around the world, countries in which animal fat consumption is high (Sweden, Denmark, Norway, Switzerland, and Belgium, for example), report higher death rates from prostate cancer compared with countries that have low animal fat consumption (Japan, Thailand, Taiwan, and the Philippines).

The possibility of some kind of protection in the low-fat Japanese diet has raised a number of hypotheses. Soy products release chemicals called isoflavones, which may be protective. Soy also reduces the level of circulating testosterone and blocks the conversion of testosterone into its more potent form, dihydrotestosterone.

Besides the protection offered by soy products, Japanese men consume more vitamin D, which is contained in the national diet of fish, and substantially smaller amounts of animal fat, since they do not eat as much red meat as North Americans, probably because it is too expensive. It is not clear at this time how much of the protection comes from consuming soy and high levels of vitamin D, and how much from avoiding juicy steaks.

Tomatoes are known to release a chemical called lycopene, which is also a protective. For maximum benefit, however, the tomatoes must be cooked in oil, which releases the important cancer-fighting lycopene.

If this appears to be an endorsement for spaghetti and pizza, so be it. Recently, lycopene has been constituted in capsule form. Several capsules a day is enough to guarantee an intake that is equivalent of a pound or two of tomatoes. A small number of prostate cancer patients have taken large doses of lycopene and have actually seen their PSA levels fall. Further, there is even early evidence that such high intakes of lycopene may inhibit the growth of cancers that are already present.

The lycopene story has yet to be fully told, however. What we surmise is that just as Japanese men have benefited from fish, so Italian men have shown lower incidence of prostate cancer – probably because of the amount of tomatoes that seem to find their way into Italian cuisine.

Men born with an enzyme deficiency so that their testosterone cannot be converted into the more powerful dihydrotestosterone do not develop prostate cancer. As this enzyme (5-alpha-reductase) can be inactivated by the drug Proscar (finasteride) or Avodart (dutasteride), it makes sense to wonder if this might not be a chemical preventative for prostate cancer. A widespread study in the United States compared the effects of Proscar versus a placebo, an inactive drug that looks identical to the real drug but which has no medicinal value. Over 18,000 men were enrolled in the study, and the results revealed a 25% reduction in prostate cancer. The reduction was definitely more in the low grade cancer, with no dramatic reduction in high grade cancer. There was even some concern that Proscar promoted high grade cancer, although most experts feel that the apparent increased risk was an artifact, that the gland shrunk by the pill made it more likely for the cancer to be diagnosed. A more recent Avodart study showed similar results: decreased rate of low grade cancer, possible heightened risk of high grade cancer.

The risk of high grade cancer has forced the pharmaceutical firms to stop promoting the 5-alpha-reductase inhibitors (Avodart or Proscar) as a cancer preventing drug. Still, in a recent study, men with low grade cancer were assigned Avodart or a placebo. Those on Avodart showed less progression.

Furthermore, a hint that Proscar might make a difference comes from the observation that men who take it show two metabolites (androstenediol glucuronide and androsterone glucuronide) that are similar to those found in Japanese men living in Japan.

Until a vaccine to prevent prostate cancer is developed, then, drugs like Proscar or Avodart, as well as lifestyle changes, genetic manipulation, and dietary supplements remain the best bets in our fight against further development of this fearsome affliction.

12

PROSTATE CANCER:
The Diagnosis

No matter how sophisticated may be the development of medical diagnostic machines, there is still nothing that can equal the skilled hand of the urologist, coupled with a profound knowledge of the prostate gland and of the symptoms described by the patient. It is in this seemingly simple procedure that the physician can determine if there is a disease to be reckoned with or whether that test, in conjunction with some blood samples, will give the patient a clean bill of health.

Back in the 1970s, the early diagnosis of prostate cancer used to depend exclusively on the rectal examination. The doctor placed his gloved and lubricated index finger into the rectum, as he or she does today, and glided it over the back surface of the prostate through the front wall of the rectum to try to feel if the gland had hardened or had formed any irregularities. In this way, enlargement could be discerned. So could a nodule or an asymmetry that might suggest a cancer.

Medical students have always been taught that the surface of the prostate gland should feel like the fleshy part of the hand, and cancer like a knuckle. Thus, when a doctor felt the equivalent of a frozen pea imbedded on the back surface of a prostate that might feel like a hard-boiled egg without its shell, he or she immediately suspected a tumour – as would still be the case – and arranged for the hard spot to be biopsied. This method of biopsy used to be done by guiding a needle into the hardened area of the prostate with a finger inserted into the rectum to remove a tiny sliver of tissue that could be sent to the laboratory for pathological examination. Sometimes the urologist performed a biopsy by actually making an incision between the scrotum and the anus under either a local or a general anaesthetic, and retrieving a sample of prostate tissue with a scalpel.

The size of the hardened area suggested whether the cancer was confined to the prostate or had spread beyond its wall. Total removal of the gland – a radical prostatectomy – was inevitably recommended when the disease was confined to the prostate. But it was considered inappropriate if it wasn't. In this case, other forms of non-surgical treatment were immediately set in motion.

One might wonder about the value of the digital rectal examination, as it is obvious that only the posterior aspect of the gland can be palpated by the examining finger. The fact is, however, that seventy percent of all prostate tumours originate in the rear of the gland, and this is the one the examining finger reaches easily.

Both the diagnostics of prostate cancer and the treatment of a tumour that was confined to the gland suddenly became a medical issue in the early 1980s when Dr. Willet Whitmore, one of North America's most highly respected urological cancer surgeons, who was also Chief of Urology at Memorial Sloan-Kettering Hospital in New York City, reviewed and reported his results of radical prostatectomies, then considered the definitive treatment for a tumour. His successes by this surgery were infrequent, he said. Many patients he thought he had cured with radical prostatectomies developed recurrent cancer some years later.

This led Dr. Whitmore to question the value of removing a man's prostate. He wondered if those patients who had been cured by this surgery might have done just as well without it. He also considered the possibility that those patients who had died of prostate cancer following a prostatectomy might not have been helped by it, either.

His famous statement, which rings like a Zen koan – "If it's

103

curable, is it necessary? And when it's necessary, is it curable?" – became known as Whitmore's conundrum. After the release of his report, many perfectly reputable urologists around the world gave up doing radical prostatectomies and referred those patients with localized cancer to their radiotherapy colleagues.

Meanwhile, it was obvious that diagnostic procedures more accurate than the index finger were needed to ascertain the extent of a tumour, and this resulted in the development of the simple blood test we know as the PSA, which changed the face of urological diagnostics.

A Buffalo clinic-cum-research centre called Roswell Park gets much of the credit for this, but, as with most scientific innovations, honours should have been distributed more widely – on a global basis, in fact. The Japanese scientist, Dr. M. Hara, first defined a protein that could liquefy the gelatinous semen. Dr. L. M. K. Chung and his colleagues were the first to show that this protein was specific to the prostate gland and named it "prostate specific antigen." Back in Buffalo, meanwhile, Dr. M. C. Wang and his associates had established the usefulness of this blood test.

Shortly afterwards, and back in Japan, Dr. Hiroki Watanabe was working diligently in his Kyoto clinic to make trans-rectal ultrasound examinations of the prostate gland meaningful, and Dr. Patrick Walsh, at Johns Hopkins, was busy clarifying the nerve bundle that he thought was responsible for retaining erection. He developed an anatomical approach to the radical prostatectomy which was the beginning of what we now call the "nerve-sparing" operation – a procedure that now enables many potent men to retain their erectile capabilities after surgery and almost all others to control their urine so they do not suffer the indignity of incontinence.

Today, most knowledgeable patients are as familiar with their PSA results as they are with their cholesterol levels, blood pressure readings, and weight fluctuations. So much so, that they have been heard to exchange them – like hockey scores or golf handicaps – in clinics across the world.

INTERPRETING THE PSA LEVEL

As we have seen, PSA is a protein that is secreted by every prostate gland cell and that is responsible for making the gelatinous ejaculate liquid. If it were a protein secreted exclusively by prostate cancer cells, it would be the perfect indicator, or marker: "If it's in the blood there's a cancer, and when it isn't, there is no cancer."

As it is, it is a reasonable marker because cancer cells secrete PSA into the bloodstream ten times more than normal prostate cells. This is not because cancer cells themselves make more PSA, but because more is likely to be released into the blood stream.

A PSA reading is a machine-generated analysis of a small amount of blood taken from the patient's forearm, where the veins are most accessible. A level of 4 nanogram per 1 ml emerged as the "magic" figure. Readings below this were, for most men, associated with prostate glands that did not harbour a cancer. Those above it were suspect. More recently, however, the enormous popularity of the "magic" 4 figure has come under criticism. Even the doctors who first suggested that it might be a critical figure, like Thomas Stamey and William Catalona, now feel that the figure was chosen without clear-cut data.

Unfortunately, twenty percent of prostate cancers are not associated with an increased release of PSA at all, and this complicates the issue as well. Furthermore, PSA readings will be higher when:

- There are more prostate cells, as in an enlarged prostate;
- The cells are irritated, as in prostatitis;
- There is a sudden loss of blood flow to a part of the prostate, causing the equivalent of a "heart attack" of the gland,

a condition known as prostatic infarct.

Guidelines that evolved related the level of a man's PSA count to his age, the size of his prostate, and how *rapidly* this count has increased over time.

In a system known as "age-adjusted" PSA, a man under fifty ideally has a reading of less than 2.5. If he is under sixty it should be less than 3.5, under seventy less than 4.5, and under eighty less than 6.5. In other words, men in these age brackets with "ideal" PSA readings may have low-level cancers that need not be treated. Conversely, they may not have cancer all.

Unfortunately, some of these men may also be among the twenty-percent whose prostate tumours are not reflected in the number of PSA-cells their prostates secrete, and they may have cancers even though the PSA count indicates otherwise.

This brings us to another kind of reading, one that is related to the density of PSA as it relates to prostate size. The dimensions of the gland are calculated by an ultrasound measurement of width, length, and height, and its volume by a simple mathematical formula. When volume is multiplied by 0.15, it denotes an acceptable PSA reading that is related directly to prostate size.

Finally, a PSA reading causes some concern if it rises by more than 0.75 units per year. Annual increases in the PSA level constitute what is called PSA velocity, and this, in my estimation, has been proven more predictive of cancer than a PSA reading based only on age or gland size. Furthermore, when the initial PSA reading is under 3.0, a rise of more than 0.5, rather than 0.75 should be considered suspect.

More recently, a further refinement in the interpretation of PSA readings has evolved – one that is designed to make them even more meaningful than they already are. This development is based on the fact that a PSA level that is not protein-bound rises with enlarged prostates, while PSA readings that are actually *bound* to protein are elevated when cancer is present – a more accurate marker. It means that while a man may indeed have a relatively high level of PSA in his blood count, and one that is free and not protein-bound, his reading will be high, but his problem may be an enlarged prostate instead of a tumour.

A fairly reliable guideline is this: A free- to total-PSA ratio of less than 0.1 usually means a high risk of cancer. If the ratio is more than 0.25, it is likely that the patient is unlikely to have cancer but has an enlarged prostate.

There is heated debate within the medical community as to whether every man beyond middle age should undergo regular PSA testing. Both the American Cancer Society and the American Urological Association say he should. They favour annual testing for all men starting at age fifty, and at age forty for those who have a family history of prostate cancer. These established medical bodies also agree that *all* African-Americans need to begin to be monitored at around age forty.

Those opposed to universal testing contend that this kind of screening will prove too expensive, will not necessarily translate into longer lives, and will create a population of disillusioned men who are upset that PSA screening led them to medical procedures that left them with problematic side effects, like incontinence and erectile dysfunction.

Where do I stand on this question? There is no doubt in my mind that PSA testing has permitted the earlier diagnosis of prostate cancer. In fact, it has been known to pick up early cancers twice as often as digital rectal examinations. I admit, however, that such widespread PSA testing has led to the removal of many more prostate glands than was necessary. All too often men have suffered some of the nasty side effects opponents to universal screening are concerned about – varying degrees of incontinence and erectile dysfunction, on the one hand, and complications with their incisions on the other.

Those same opponents also claim that indiscriminate PSA testing has sent men into ill-advised and drastic surgery from which they have died, but on this point I must set the record straight. The number of deaths from prostate surgery of any kind – including radical prostatectomies – has declined drastically over the years to such a point that they are now almost unheard of. Further, in the same period, the death rate from prostate cancer itself has dropped to a similar extent, and this has been due directly to the very things those opponents have opposed – widespread PSA tests as an early method of diagnosing cancer.

I have had one post-operative death among roughly two thousand procedures I have carried out. The patient, who happened to be the father of a colleague, an orthopaedic surgeon, had a fatal pulmonary embolus, a blood clot that had formed in his pelvic vein and migrated to his heart.

While some dissenters claim that the drop in prostate cancer deaths is directly related to lower levels of animal fats found in our foods, I must take issue once again. The death rate has fallen most dramatically in those parts of Canada and the United States where radical prostatectomies are carried out as a matter of routine for younger men with proven prostate cancer. Indeed, I honestly believe that early diagnosis translates into higher rates of cure, and that PSA screening contributes to this success. So, I must reinforce my point – that every man should have an annual PSA test and an annual digital rectal examination from the age of forty or fifty, depending on his family history and ethnic background.

Annual rectal examinations and PSA tests for all men aged between fifty and seventy, and even younger for those with a family history of prostate cancer, were once supported by the Canadian Urological Association. That was until the organization's executive changed its mind, deciding that there was no hard evidence that such universal testing could be justified, and recommending PSA testing only for men with prostate-related symptoms and for those who asked for it.

There is a covert suggestion in the Association's recommendation that if a man has no symptoms, he is unlikely to have prostate cancer, and, as we now know, this is far from the truth. My colleagues and I have seen numerous patients who delayed PSA testing because they had no symptoms, and who were shocked to find their levels severely elevated when they finally had it done. On biopsy, many of these men had advanced cancer and angrily asked why the PSA testing had been discouraged. I had no good answer for them.

The second aspect of the recommendation that suggests testing only for "those men are concerned about prostate cancer" begs the questions: "Who isn't concerned about prostate cancer?" Or, "Who shouldn't be concerned about it?"

Is this policy an attempt by the Association to restrict PSA testing to the more-aware elitist population? I think the Association should rethink its stance.

Once and for all: Statistics show that the early detection of prostate cancer through early and regular PSA testing has – even though prostate cancer is generally slow-growing – saved and improved many more lives than it has spoiled or ended.

The controversy over universal PSA testing was revived in 2011 when a US advisory board declared that there was not enough evidence to encourage universal screening. The arguments put forward were as follows:

1. Ultrasound-guided biopsies have not been free of complications. Some of these complications were even fatal;
2. Studies on the merits of screening do show an increase in lives saved, but the numbers are not impressive. Something

like 40 prostatectomies must be done to show one extra life
saved;

3. There is overdiagnosis and overtreatment of prostate cancer.

In refuting these claims, let me draw an analogy with maintaining the life of your automobile. Will your car last longer with
regular check-ups – or with service only when there is a problem?
I would argue that in the hands of a good and honest mechanic,
your car will last longer with regular check-ups. In the hands of an
incompetent and dishonest mechanic, your car may not last as long.

Complications from prostate cancer can and do occur, but using
that as an argument is like arguing that you should not purchase a
car because you could get injured in an automobile accident.

To argue that not enough lives have been saved by radical prostatectomy is like arguing that not enough lives have been saved by
seat belts. Should we abandon them because they save a life only
once in every forty accidents?

Finally, what is overdiagnosis of prostate cancer? If the cancer is
there, should it not be diagnosed? I can understand overtreatment
of prostate cancer, but I don't understand the concept of overdiagnosis. At this time we cannot predict which relatively low grade
cancer will stay dormant and which will progress. We know that
roughly 30% will progress, but we cannot claim to know that we
can always react appropriately in time to effect a cure. Dr. Lawrence
Klotz, who has been a strong proponent of careful monitoring of
low grade cancer, reported that when he eventually took some of
these men to surgery, 25% had positive margins, that is, cancer at
the edges of the specimen, and 8% had cancer in the lymph nodes.
Wouldn't these patients have been better off with earlier intervention? Was it not opportunity lost?

I think the concern for overtreatment of prostate cancer is appropriate. Certainly a man with a slight elevation in his PSA, let's

say to a level of 5.5 and a 12 core biopsy that showed one core with a Gleason 6 cancer is best followed. But, what if his PSA rises to 7.2, and two cores are now positive a year later? Should we wait until half the cores are positive and the cancer occupies more than fifty per cent of all the cores ? Although there is a movement to re-name the Gleason 6 cancer an "adenosis" rather than a "carcinoma" I feel more comfortable advising my patients with any progression to seek active treatment, such as ablative surgery or radiotherapy.

The American Urological Association guideline committee responded to the suggestion that PSA screening may be more harmful than helpful with a position statement in 2013. They suggest that apart from men predisposed, such as African-Americans, or those with a family history, PSA screening should start at age fifty-five and stop at age sixty-nine, and occur every two years rather than annually.

I disagree. The recommendation to curtail PSA testing was not because a better marker has been developed. I favour initial testing when a man is in his forties, annual testing and biopsy if the initial reading is over 3, and annual screening after age fifty to be continued indefinitely. Withholding the test at age seventy is insulting to healthy men sufficiently concerned about their health. Overtreatment will remain a problem until we can better distinguish those who will progress from those who will not; but, I believe it is better to err on the side of overtreatment than undertreatment.

ULTRASOUND IMAGING

When the PSA reading is out of the normal range, and/or if the rectal examination has revealed a prostatic abnormality that suggests a tumour, ultrasound imaging comes into play. It is widely used to ascertain if a biopsy is warranted.

Fishermen use ultrasound to detect the presence of fish. Gynaecologists use it to discern any abnormal development of the fetus, or its sex if the parents wish to know. Kidney stones can be located with ultrasound and assessed in terms of their size and the degree of blockage they are causing within the urinary tract. Suspicious lumps on such organs as the liver and the kidneys can be categorized by ultrasound and diagnosed as being either cancerous tumours or more innocent fluid-filled cysts. Damaged blood vessels, like an aneurysm, can be assessed by ultrasound, too, so that a specialist may be able to decide on ways to replace or repair them.

Ultrasound imaging of the prostate gland with a rectal probe has come a long way since Dr. Watanabe got his patients to sit on an erect probe in his Kyoto clinic more than thirty years ago. His first efforts initially showed no more than a few bumps on the surface of the prostate that suggested asymmetry and nothing else. But it was a start, and one that showed how sound waves could be used in urology to wonderful advantage.

The human ear hears sound waves of between twenty and twenty-thousand vibrations per second, and dogs far more. Today, however, ultrasound equipment is much more sophisticated and can bounce a higher number of sound waves – seven million vibrations a second, in fact – that no animal could ever hope to hear.

More important is that it can "see" well inside a gland as the waves bounce off fat, glandular tissue, muscle, and cancerous tissue differently, and the results of this can be made to form images on a television screen that are invaluable to specialists like radiologists, obstetricians, and urologists.

The degree of echogenicity – that is, the "bounce" of the ultrasound waves off different types of tissue – has a characteristic pattern. Thus the image obtained on the screen depicts clearly the contour of the prostate gland because the bounce of surrounding fat is quite different from the bounce from solid tissue. Adjacent structures like the seminal vesicles, urethra, and bladder are also clearly delineated.

The prostate gland itself is projected onto the screen as a mottled grey organ, with the inner part easily distinguishable from the outer part. Within the outer part there may be areas that look darker – or hypoechoeic – or lighter, hyperechoeic.

Tumours show up on an ultrasound screen most often as dark spots, or hypoechoeic areas. Some cancers, however, are grey and some light. Whatever their textures, they are usually quite discernible to the urologist and are invaluable in helping him or her decide the next step in the management of suspected prostate cancer.

For several decades now, an elevated PSA count, an unacceptable increase in the PSA count (acceleration), or an abnormal rectal examination led to an ultrasound and ultrasound-guided biopsies of the prostate. This paradigm has been challenged by magnetic resonance imaging (MRI) of the prostate as a prelude to biopsy. Considerable expertise is required for proper interpretation of the MRI images, but there is little doubt that the technology represents a major innovation and will play an increasingly meaningful role in the future.

13

PROSTATE CANCER:
The Biopsy, and When it is Positive

Fifty years ago, a diagnosis of prostate cancer spelled the beginning of the end for the patient. Although radical prostatectomies went a long way toward mitigating the final result, the unfortunate truth was that the survival rate was not what we see today, given the updated diagnostic tools we have at hand.

Nevertheless, the psychological and emotional effects of such a diagnosis merited understanding, information, and encouragement to the patient involved. Today, the diagnosis may mean many more years of healthy, happy life; however, one cannot underestimate the importance of psychological as well as medical support for the long-term benefit of the patient. Indeed, his outlook on life may go a long way toward supporting him in the odyssey which lies ahead. For this reason, urologists now underscore the fact that one must deal with the whole patient and not only the disease process.

With the help of modern technology, urologists are now able to not only capture images of organs on their screens, but use them to ensure more accurate biopsies than those done twenty years ago, and at a first attempt.

Ultrasound is absolutely invaluable when the need arises for a definitive biopsy – not to show pictures or shapes of the prostate this time, but to help a specialist penetrate a tumour with a biopsy needle. Sound waves can show a target at which a biopsy needle must be aimed, and it's a bull's eye every time because ultrasound also guides the way.

When biopsies are performed, the needles are directed not only at the suspicious areas, but evenly into other regions, too. This is to ensure that the entire gland is being carefully scrutinized for cancer.

Needle one goes into the apex of the left side of the prostate, needle three into the outer mid-body on the gland's left side, and needle five into the left base close to the bladder. Needles two, four, and six go into corresponding areas on the right side of the prostate.

These six biopsies are made by lining up the dots seen on the screen, which indicate where the needle will traverse, and firing the spring loaded gun into the dots' path. The needle is shot in with such speed that there is no stretching of tissue, which is the main cause of pain. Needles driven in slowly, as was the case with that finger-directed biopsy, stretch tissue and make for a very painful procedure.

What we now call trans-rectal ultrasound-guided needle biopsies thus allow precise, multiple, and less painful biopsies than was the case thirty years ago.

The standard six cores have been replaced by the new standard ten or twelve cores. When ten cores are taken, an extra one slightly more medial is taken at the base and mid-portion of the gland on each side to make ten. Two more medial cores at the apex make twelve. Saturation biopsies – where many more cores are taken depending upon the size of the gland – have been largely abandoned.

Patients are prepared for the biopsy with antibiotics starting the evening before the test which are continued for two days after it. Lower bowel clean out with an enema used to be routine just before the biopsy, but this has since been abandoned as being unnecessary and with no adverse outcomes.

Antibiotics, usually Ciprofloxacin for three days starting the night before, prevents infections most of the time. In up to three per cent of cases, however, there can be serious infections requiring hospitalization and intravenous antibiotics. In an effort to reduce this serious morbidity, some centres have insisted upon anal swabs with sensitivity testing beforehand, or stronger courses of intramuscular or intravenous antibiotics at the time of biopsy. Whether these regimes have proven their worth is not certain. In my own practice, I ask my patients if they have taken antibiotics during the past year. If they have, I give them an intramuscular shot of gentamicin 80 mg one hour before the biopsy. I am debating whether I should extend this regime to men who are hospital workers.

For the actual procedure, the patient is told to lie on his side, curled up in the foetal position, with his knees as close as possible to his chest. A finger examination of his prostate is done first, and this will lubricate and dilate the passage in preparation to receive the probe, which is wider than any finger. Measurements of the prostate are taken at this time, and a thorough ultrasound examination follows. This takes no more than a few minutes.

The needle-loaded gun for the biopsy is placed in the shaft that runs through the probe, and the patient is instructed not to move. The gun is fired when the directing dots line up – where the biopsy needle must traverse in order to get a meaningful sample. The needle is then withdrawn, but not the probe, and the process is repeated. The needle is re-inserted for the other biopsies.

Bleeding from the needle sites is usually minimal, but on rare occasions it can be quite significant. I have not been impressed with any quick measures to lessen this, such as applying finger pressure to the prostate through the rectum. In any case, bleeding following a biopsy is always temporary. Those patients who have been on such blood-thinners such as Aspirin, and anti-coagulation drugs such as Coumadin or Plavix, are told to stop taking them for about a week (or two for Plavix) before undergoing a prostatic biopsy.

When the gland is particularly large, some prostate centres recommend more than ten biopsy needles. This makes sense, though in my experience, ten is quite enough. Most patients are relieved when the gun is fired for the last time, and they would be most reluctant to agree to more needles. When the procedure must be repeated — because of a further and unacceptable rise in the PSA level, for example — patients agree to the test somewhat reluctantly.

A number of patients ask if I can give them a local anaesthetic. Sometimes I comply, but I often advise against it. For most men, the most distressing part of the test is the insertion of the probe, and there is no way to freeze the passage. I can freeze for the needles, but I may be increasing the risks of infection, I tell them. Patients who have undergone the biopsy with or without the local tell me they discern little or no difference. I do prescribe sub-lingual Ativan 1 mg before the procedure for extra nervous candidates.

When patients are reluctant to subject themselves to repeated biopsies, as they often are, I do something I think might help them. One of my younger patients, a school teacher, bears witness to this. He was fifty-six when he first had an ultrasound-guided biopsy. His PSA score was 5.2, which was high for a man of his age, but the biopsy itself was negative. One year later, however, his PSA was 7.6, and he underwent another biopsy. This was also negative for cancer.

On his own volition, and against my advice, he skipped a year and returned to see me when his PSA score had reached 9.2. A third biopsy was also negative, but a year after this, his PSA had soared to 10.7.

Another ultrasound and biopsy was recommended, but the patient declined it. He'd had enough of the needles, he said, and was willing to take his chances with fate.

I understood this perfectly and felt we might try something else a little more comfortable. Even though he'd had no problems with his urine flow, I persuaded the man to take Proscar (finasteride) and it worked. Six months later his PSA was 6.3 — forty percent lower!

We agreed the patient should have another PSA in six months, and, if the level had dropped by another ten percent, I would consider it unlikely that we were dealing with cancer at all. I have made this recommendation in similar circumstances a few times since, and those patients unfortunate enough to have had positive ultrasound-guided biopsies are extremely grateful for it.

Now, I have an understanding with these men. We will only agree to further biopsies if, after having taken Proscar, the PSA has not dropped by pre-determined amounts – by forty percent after six months, or by fifty percent after one year.

This way of following patients with rising PSA has been modified by progress made in magnetic resonance imaging (MRI) of the prostate. This diagnostic test can pick up lesions in the anterior part of the gland, an area not clearly delineated by trans-rectal ultrasound. Biopsy of the suspicious area, anterior or not, can be done with higher expectation of positive results. MRI before biopsy may indeed represent a paradigm shift in the management of prostate cancer.

THE BIOPSY RESULT

I would be remiss if I did not elaborate here on the role of the pathologist. In urology, as in most other medical disciplines, he or she is indispensable.

A pathologist is a medical doctor who has spent a minimum of five years in specialized training after medical school and has qualified as an expert by passing stringent examinations. The pathologist is often asked, by all manner of hospital doctors, to examine tissue samples and render an opinion on what may be wrong with them. By touch, by sight, or by closer scrutiny under a microscope, he or she can make a valuable pronouncement on the presence or absence of all kinds of diseases, their nature, and their seriousness.

When it comes to urology, pathology is a vital link in the chain of treatments that the medical team may have prescribed to any one of their patients. Pathologists do a particularly admirable job for us because they are the final arbiters in defining prostate cancer. When a pathologist is asked to rule prostate cancer either in or out, he is, in effect, basing an opinion entirely on those little slivers of tissue the urologist has sent him — pieces of flesh that resemble ten lengths of thread, each about a centimetre long.

Almost without exception, the pathologist's biopsy results are returned from the laboratory within a week or two, although it is possible to have the tissue processed within hours or days. The pathologist's report will indicate one of several findings:

- Negative – no cancer;
- The presence of what is called **PIN** – prostatic intraepithelial neoplasia – which means that the biopsy has detected some tissue changes that indicate cancer may develop later;
- Evidence of what is called small acinar proliferation, considered slightly more ominous than PIN as a precancerous change;
- Positive – the absolute presence of cancer.

There are, however, some other elements to consider. Negative biopsies may show changes associated with an enlarged prostate, or even prostatitis. In the ultrasound, prostatitis is never clearly indicated, but is more definitely proven in the biopsy, when inflammatory cells are seen by the pathologist to have invaded the prostate.

You may ask why the biopsy isn't automatically done to detect prostatitis. The answer is really quite simple: it would too often be hit or miss. That is to say, the urologist would not know where to steer his needle in his search for prostatitis, because the ultrasound would not provide him with a path. So, when prostatitis is found during biopsy, the needle has made a serendipitous discovery, which is nonetheless useful. As I have indicated before, a prostatic abscess alters the ultrasound image sufficiently to help establish the diagnosis.

It is more important to remember here that while low grade PIN has almost no significance, high grade PIN or acinar proliferation can be premalignant.

The distinction between low grade and high grade PIN, by the way, is a tricky problem for pathologists. I have had slides designated high grade by one pathologist and low grade by another. When this controversy occurs in the midst of a rising PSA it can provoke enormous anxiety for the patient, and it is left to me to reiterate the bottom line as I have come to know it – that perhaps twenty-five percent of all patients with high grade PINs eventually develop prostate cancer.

One of my patients, a colleague physician, is walking testimony to the confusion – not to mention the anguish – that a high grade PIN can provoke. He was forty-six when he first came to see me, after having run a routine PSA blood test on himself, of all things. He was alarmed when the biochemistry laboratory told him it was 6.4. He was certain he had cancer.

My ultrasound-guided biopsy on him, however, revealed only a high grade PIN, but another PSA blood test done at the hospital six months later indicated a reading of 7.2! His PSA was rising. A repeat biopsy was arranged, and again the results for cancer were negative, though two of the six biopsy specimens still showed a high grade PIN. At this point, I had the slides reviewed by Dr. Jonathan Epstein at Johns Hopkins, a recognized authority on PIN. He felt that a high grade PIN had been too strong a diagnosis and that the patient's grade really bordered on being low.

The patient, meanwhile, was so preoccupied with the possibility that he had cancer that he was no longer able to work. He thought this was inevitable, so he asked me to remove his prostate. There was no indication that such drastic surgery was needed, I said, but I might accede to his wishes if he gave me explicit consent. He did.

Later, when I reviewed his chart, I suspected that he would almost certainly develop cancer later anyway, and was probably better off having the surgery now than when he was older – particularly since his state of mind had been so adversely distorted by his obsession that he was jeopardizing his marriage and his career.

Two years after first seeing this man, I performed the operation. The pathology report on the removed prostate revealed the presence of a high grade PIN, but there were still no signs of cancer. Nonetheless, the patient never regretted having had the operation, and fortunately he suffered no major side effects. He is potent and dry.

THE PIN REPORT

Assessing PIN is a relatively new way pathologists have agreed to define cell changes in the biopsy specimens urologists have sent them. The technique they use entails putting slices of the same specimens they have used for cancer under a microscope. Once they are convinced that cancer is absent, they look for fragmentation of the basement membrane – the tell-tale sign of PIN.

More important for you to remember is that if repeat biopsies are negative, careful follow-up is still necessary, and with regular or semi-annual PSA tests.

SMALL ACINAR PROLIFERATION

The designation "small acinar proliferation" is considered more ominous today than high grade PIN. Under the microscope the pathologist is seeing more glands, but no nuclear changes associated with cancer. When the nuclear changes of cancer are present, the images are like that of Gleason Grade one cancer, which is characterized by more acini or glands.

THE GLEASON GRADE

While the biopsy indicates the presence of cancer, other information is required to determine its type, character, and severity. This brings us to what is called the Gleason Grade, so called because it was devised by an American pathologist named Dr. Donald Gleason more than twenty-five years ago. Since then it has become the international standard by which prostate cancer is measured and described.

To put this another way: prostate cancer is reported in terms of the Gleason Grade, which is a score between two and ten. The pathologist may also report the percentage of cancer involved within the tiny cylinder of tissue he has been sent to examine. So, the Gleason Grade is really a pathologist's opinion of the degree of differentiation in cancer cells, and it is one that influences the urologist's plan of action.

Coupled with the PSA, the Gleason Grade gives a urologist the most valuable information he or she requires to be able to arrive at a prognosis. Once the seriousness of cancer and the extent to which it may have spread are known – the stage of the disease – the proper way to manage it can be assigned.

The degree of cell-differentiation is the key to how well a patient is likely to fare with the disease. Usually, one who has a well-differentiated tumour will do better than one who has a poorly differentiated tumour.

Obviously, there is no point in removing a patient's prostate gland without removing all of his cancer, so it's important to determine if surgery is the answer to his problems or whether he might be better served by other treatment. Before we can do this, we must study the Gleason Grade carefully. Its goal, after all, is to help ascertain which cancer will need immediate treatment because it is spreading, with what available techniques it should be treated, and whether it will need immediate treatment at all.

HOW THE PATHOLOGIST ASSIGNS THE GLEASON GRADE

The pathologist determines the presence of prostate cancer when he sees changes in the appearance of certain cells. Cancer cells have a more variegated nucleus than ordinary, healthy cells. That is to say, they are not uniform in their sizes, shapes, and clusters. Also they show prominent disfiguration within the nucleus itself. Pathologists determine this information by seeing how clusters of cells stain differently than normal cells.

Furthermore, as cells divide more quickly when they have been replaced by cancer cells, cancer can be readily detected when these cells are stained.

Perhaps I may make the Gleason Grade more comprehensible by suggesting an analogy between the pathological grading and the box of raspberries. If you can imagine prostate tissue under the microscope looking rather like a box of freshly picked raspberries lying among leaves and twigs, you might be able to understand what a thin cross-section of such a box might look like. Different raspberries would be cut in different places so that more or less of their central cavities will be seen. Some will be cut at their tips, others at their bases, some in cross-sections, others obliquely.

The term the pathologist uses to describe the raspberries is *acini,* cell clusters so shaped that they each have a central cavity. These are the raspberries. The twigs and leaves, meanwhile, are the supporting tissue, which the pathologist calls *stroma*.

A Gleason 1 cancer rating is assigned when there are more berries – or cell clusters – relative to the amount of twigs, or stroma, in the box. This is what pathologists call "a decreased amount of stroma." In this case, there are no berries – or cell clusters – stuck together. Nor do the berries, or cell clusters, vary in size. More berries! Does that not remind us of small acinar proliferation?

A Gleason Grade 2 cancer rating is assigned when the raspberries – or cell clusters – are of different sizes. This is not to be confused with berries cut high or low, giving an appearance of different sizes. A slice of a box of raspberries of different sizes should be distinguishable from one with uniform size. In pathological terms, this would be described as "variation in glandular size or variation in size of acini."

Gleason Grade 3 cancer describes a situation where three or four raspberries – or cell clusters – have come together, and are not just lying adjacent to one another but are actually stuck together. The berries, or cell clusters, are so well bonded that the hairs on them at the point of contact are undetectable. The pathological equivalent of the hair on the raspberries is cytokeratin. When the pathologist stains for the cytokeratin and can't see it, the glands or acini have coalesced.

Gleason Grade 4 cancer describes the situation when four or more berries coalesce, and the descriptive term pathologists use for this is "cribriform pattern of invasive cancer." In our box of raspberries, this would signify the further loss of hair so that four or more berries appear joined.

Gleason Grade 5 cancer has the appearance of a slice of a box of raspberries that has been stepped upon. Any evidence of the hollow part of the berry is lost. Almost all of the fruit has been completely crushed.

THE GLEASON GRADE

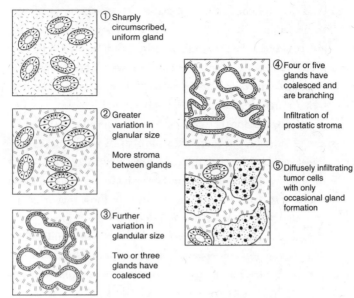

① Sharply circumscribed, uniform gland

② Greater variation in glanular size

More stroma between glands

③ Further variation in glandular size

Two or three glands have coalesced

④ Four or five glands have coalesced and are branching

Infiltration of prostatic stroma

⑤ Diffusely infiltrating tumor cells with only occasional gland formation

In assigning the Gleason Grade, the pathologist takes the two most predominant patterns seen under his microscope and adds them together. If, for example, he sees no more than two to three raspberries joined together, he safely determines this to mean Grade 3. If he sees no other pattern – such as more berries joining – he calls it 3 plus 3, meaning a Gleason 6, and so on down the line.

The pathologist uses a few tricks to clarify confusing scenarios. If, for instance, he is not sure if he is looking at a prostate cell, he can stain for PSA. If the cell picks up the PSA, it has to be a prostate cell. Also, when he is not certain if the acini are merely touching, or coalescing, he can stain for the equivalent of the hairs on the berries. This is the cytokeratin stain which, when absent, suggests the presence of cancer with all its invasive features.

From this description it should be apparent that the subtle difference lies in distinguishing Gleason Grade 3 from Gleason Grade 4, and this is indeed the distinction that may be the most significant.

Cancer patients often ask me, somewhat hopefully, if the pathologist could have been mistaken in his opinion. Could he have diagnosed a cancerous tumour when there wasn't one? This, I explain, is possible; pathologists are human, after all. It does not happen often, though. In fact, it rarely happens at all.

It is also possible for the slides of one person to be mistaken for the slides of another, but there are a number of safeguards to protect against such accidents, and for the most part these work well.

From the urologist's standpoint, Gleason Grades of 6 and lower are considered to denote low grade tumours or those that are slow-growing – the "pussy cat." Grades 8, 9, and 10 are considered to depict high grade aggressive tumours – the "tiger." Gleason Grade 7, meanwhile, is categorized separately as an entity unto itself because it could probably have been either a 6 or an 8. As should be apparent a Gleason 7 that is 4+3 is worse than a Gleason 7 that is 3+4.

STAGING

When a patient has been diagnosed with prostate cancer with a pathological level of differentiation that has been reflected by the Gleason Grade, the next stage is a series of evaluations aimed at determining the extent of his cancer. This is a process called staging, and it is done in one of two ways:

- The ABC method, which dates back to the 1960s;
- The TNM method, which was introduced in 1992.

Because the TNM method is the more widely accepted form today, I will describe it here with the ABC equivalent in parenthesis.

- T1a (A1) means that the tumour was found by chance in the prostate tissue removed by a trans-urethral resection (TURP) and that it occupies less than five percent of tissue excised during surgery;
- T1b (A2) means that more than five percent of the excised tissue is cancerous;
- T1c (A3) means that cancer was found on needle biopsy done because the PSA was elevated, not because it was suspicious on rectal examination;
- T2a (B1) means that a tumour was suspected on digital rectal examination, but that it is confined to less than one half of one lobe;
- T2b (B2) means that cancer was suspicious on digital rectal examination and involves more than half of one lobe;
- T2c (B3) means that the cancer has spread to both lobes;
- T3a (C1) means the cancer has spread outside the capsule on one side;
- T3b (C2) means that the cancer has spread beyond the capsule on both sides;
- T3c means the cancer has spread to one or both seminal vesicles;
- T4 means the cancer has spread to adjacent tissue like the bladder neck or urethra.

In advanced staging, when the cancer has spread beyond the prostate – first into the lymph nodes and later into bones and other organs – we use other designations:

- N0 means there is no lymph node involvement;
- Nx means the nodes cannot or have not been evaluated;
- N1 means that cancer is present, but that the involved node (or nodes) has (have) enlarged it by less than 2 cm;

- N2 means that cancer has enlarged one or more nodes by more than 2 cm. (The ABC method calls all these categories D1.)
- M means that there is widespread cancer, probably now in the bones;
- M0 means no distant metastases;
- Mx means distant metastases have not, and cannot, be evaluated;
- M1 means distant metastases;
- M1a means cancer has spread into nodes other than the regional nodes;
- M1b means that the cancer has spread to the bones;
- M1c means cancer has reached sites other than the skeleton, such as the liver.

(In the ABC equivalent, each of these latter categories is designated as D2 .)

BONE SCANS AND OTHERS

When we are fairly certain that the cancer has spread beyond the prostate, we must find out where it has gone, exactly, and how far it has spread. Ninety percent of the time, cancer that spreads from the prostate into the lymph nodes enters the bone, so the bone scan is absolutely imperative in helping us further define the extent of the disease.

(It would be wonderful if urologists had a test that showed whether or not cancer had invaded the lymph nodes themselves, but short of surgical exploration there are, as yet, no other accurate methods.)

A bone scan used to be routine before treatment in every prostate patient. Recently, though, it has been suggested that it is unnecessary when the Gleason Grade is under 7 and the PSA reading is under 10. I agree with this.

The bone scan for cancer begins with an intravenous injection of a radioactive material that goes directly to the skeleton. Three hours later, the patient is scanned from head to toe, a procedure that takes about one hour. The radioactive material emits gamma rays that produce the equivalent of an X-ray picture of the bones. When cancer is present, the affected areas show up as dark spots.

Some centres insist upon a CT scan as well as a bone scan for every prostate cancer patient. The CT scan can detect lymph nodes which have been enlarged by more than one centimetre in either length or width, which immediately raises the suspicion of cancer. But that is all. The problem is that nodes that are smaller than this can be cancerous, too. So a CT does not always help in defining the extent of the disease.

Cancerous changes within the prostate gland itself cannot be detected either by a CT scan. Consequently, I don't consider the CT scan helpful in staging this disease at all, but radio-oncologists consider it mandatory before treatment is begun. The configuration of the gland helps them decide how many treatments from how many directions are necessary.

It should now be apparent that once prostate cancer has been diagnosed, it is not a simple case of "on with the surgery." Far from it. What kind of treatment is best for which patient will ultimately depend on age, general health, attitude, or a combination of all three – and the kind and extent of the cancer we are trying to contain.

14

PROSTATE CANCER:
Managing the Disease

"Get it out! Get it out, and now!" are words that I hear more frequently than one would expect. Most patients, when they receive a diagnosis of prostate cancer, are ready and willing to have the offending tissue immediately removed, thus, in their eyes, ensuring a long, happy and cancer-free life for themselves. Ah, if it were only that simple and straightforward. Surgery is indeed one avenue we can use for treatment; however, there are a multitude of factors which can help us to determine if this is the best medical course of action.

No urologist wants to subject a prostate cancer patient to a radical prostatectomy unless it is going to achieve its ends. Sometimes, though, there is little choice. A relatively young, healthy man with "the tiger" must obviously have aggressive treatment. But then, must a young man with "the pussycat" be similarly treated because three in ten will progress and his cancer may become less curable later? The common argument is that there should be more than ten years' further life expectancy before settling on a procedure like a radical prostatectomy.

That is a judgment call that is not always easy to make nor necessarily accurate. It is just as difficult as determining which low grade cancer will progress and which will not. Consider an analogy to coronary artery disease. Suppose you are told that tests indicate coronary artery disease. There is a thirty percent chance of progression: corrective surgery (bypass) can be done with a chance of a cure, but there is a ten percent chance of dying from the operation. How many will want the surgery? How many would rather risk progression?

For older men who might not be able to withstand such major surgery as a radical prostatectomy, alternative treatment plans must be mapped out. These are usually done with one important factor in mind – that because prostate cancer is nearly always slow-growing, many of these patients will live out the rest of their lives with it, and without too many ill-effects.

In other words, why let treatment affect the well-being of a perfectly active seventy-five-year-old man when his condition can be contained, and to some extent improved, with what we call palliative treatment? Indeed, most such patients will eventually die from other causes and not from prostate cancer at all.

Generally, speaking there are seven ways to go, but when to apply them can be complex. Some treatments are considered curative on their own, while others are merely palliative. Also, one treatment may be more successful when it has followed another or when it is combined with another. Other procedures, however, as I will explain, are futile even when they are applied sequentially.

Prostate cancer treatments are:

- Watchful waiting or active surveillance;
- Radical prostatectomy;
- Radiotherapy;
- Combination therapy;
- Hormone therapy;
- Focal therapy;
- Experimental therapy.

The term "watchful waiting" is being displaced by the term "active surveillance," which suggests a more careful follow-up.

"Watchful waiting" usually means doing nothing until the patient develops symptoms or has complaints, which usually signify progression of the disease.

"Active surveillance," on the other hand, usually means specific measures like PSA every six months and trans-rectal biopsies of the prostate every twelve months.

WATCHFUL WAITING

During this period of observation – intense or otherwise, again depending on age or the severity of the problem – the patient is monitored to make sure that his urinary tract continues to function, and for signs that his cancer is not becoming life-threatening.

Does this period of watchful waiting, or no treatment for the disease, make any sense?

Decades ago, Swedish experts thought it did. They felt that if prostate cancer was slow-growing, as it so often is, and that many men died with it rather than from it, why not simply follow men diagnosed with the disease and offer treatment only if and when they began to suffer, from pain, perhaps, or from voiding difficulties.

Around the world, this became the accepted option when patients were elderly, usually beyond the age of seventy-five, or for men with fewer than ten years of further life expectancy. With watchful waiting, however, it became apparent that those men with high Gleason Grade cancers did poorly. Their disease advanced quickly, necessitating hormone treatment.

Might they have been better off being treated earlier, upon diagnosis? There was no clear-cut message in the medical literature on this point. In fact, the feeling was to withhold any treatment if men were symptom-free – and to delay the deployment of guns, so to speak, until it became necessary to use them. Why waste the ammunition? It may run out by the time it is really needed. The idea

132

was based on speculation, not science.

To prove this point, a team of British doctors carried out a study on older men who had advanced prostate cancer that was causing them no symptoms. Half the men were treated upon diagnosis, and the other half treated only when they developed pain. The group that was offered early treatment fared far better. They did not suffer collapsed spines caused by the invasion of cancer as often as those on whom treatment was not immediately initiated. Their urinary tracts remained unobstructed for longer. Their times to further disease, and their times to death, were also delayed. In other words, watchful waiting made very little sense.

Something should be done to help men such as these as soon as they are diagnosed. I know this from experience with a seventy-year-old man who was referred to me with a PSA reading of 8.4, but who had no difficulty urinating at all. Upon my rectal examination, his prostate was suspicious for cancer on the left side, and ultrasound-guided biopsies later revealed Gleason Grades 7 and 8 prostate cancer in three of six needle cores. The bone scan, however, was negative.

I strongly advised hormone treatment to be followed by radio-therapy – combination treatment – but the patient elected watchful waiting as had been suggested by those Swedish experts. Perhaps his decision was influenced by his ethnic origin, for he himself was Swedish. There was no way I could get him to change his mind.

One year later, his PSA had risen to 12.8, and it was only then that he agreed to the treatment I had first suggested. Soon, his PSA dropped to 2.0, but a year later it rose to 38.9. Now, a bone scan revealed metastatic lesions in his hips and ribs.

I am sad to report that further treatment failed this man. He managed at home until about six years from the time of his diagnosis, and was then admitted to hospital for palliative care until he died some weeks later. The year he'd spent in watchful waiting, to my mind, cost him his life.

I am much happier to record those occasions when watchful waiting was a more appropriate measure, as in the case of a sixty-three-year-old business man on whom I had performed a routine TURP for enlarged prostate that was causing sufficient discomfort. A Gleason Grade 6 cancer, however, was found in several chips that were sent to the laboratory after his surgery.

When I first disclosed the pathology report to the man, he wanted his prostate removed immediately. "There's no way I can live with the thought of cancer in my body," he said, which is a common reaction.

I told him his PSA reading of only 2.4 was a fairly low count and nothing to worry about. "Why don't we follow the situation with regular PSAs and rectal exams," I suggested. "There's time enough for surgery should the situation change." Besides, I added, there was no guarantee I could preserve his potency, which is something I would be concerned about if I were in his shoes.

I have followed this patient for more than ten years now, and there has been no detectable progression in his disease, nor PSA elevations, nor a deterioration in his well-being. He is a happy man.

His is not an isolated case. I have a number of men whose early cancer was discovered on prostatic chips removed because of obstructive symptoms from an enlarged prostate. Some had aggressive cancer in more than a few chips and were subjected to total removal of their gland.

Patients who elect simply to have their situations followed, rather than be treated from the outset, provide us with figures that document their risk of developing more serious complications:

- A man with a Gleason Grade 2, 3, or 4 tumour has a two percent chance of having his cancer spread each year.
- When the Gleason Grade is 5, 6, or 7, the risks climb to more than five percent annually.

- A Gleason Grade of between 7 and 10 means that the chances of developing metastases is nearly fourteen percent per year.

Dr. Alan W. Partin of the Johns Hopkins Medical Center has constructed a table that predicts the probability of prostate cancer being confined to the gland based on Gleason Grade and the PSA reading. For example:

- If a man has a Gleason score of 7, a PSA reading of 8, and non-palpable disease on rectal examination (T1C disease), his chances of having a tumour confined to his prostate is fifty percent.
- If the Gleason Grade is the same, and the PSA reading is between 10 and 20, the chances of the disease being confined to the gland drops to thirty-five percent.
- If, with the same Gleason Grade, the PSA score is above 20, the chances drop to eighteen percent. This means that there is an eighty-two percent chance that surgery alone may not cure his problem.

Dr. Partin's table, known simply as the Partin Table, is a useful guide, but decisions on what treatments should be, based on his calculations, are less straightforward. Some men will choose surgery even though, according to Dr. Partin, they have only a twenty-percent chance of a complete cure, while others with a nearly eighty-percent chance of eliminating cancer with surgery will decline it.

Many men like to make choices for themselves, while others leave them entirely to their doctors or their families. It is never an easy decision.

Of course, if watchful waiting fails and the disease worsens, the urological team must then order more conventional treatment – and soon.

ACTIVE SURVEILLANCE

Active surveillance has become more popular in recent years with better definition of the disease. The D'Amico classification is widely accepted in defining three categories of prostate cancer:

- Low risk: those with a PSA of 10 or less, Gleason Grade of 6 or less, with disease not palpable or suspicious only on one side;
- Intermediate risk: those with a PSA count between 10 and 20, Gleason grade of 7, and disease palpable on both sides and even extending to the outer margins of the prostate;
- High risk: those with a PSA higher than 20, Gleason grade of 8-10, and palpable disease beyond the extent of the gland.

The so-called "tiger" with its Gleason grade of 8 or more, is further defined by an initial PSA of 20 or more, PSA rising more than 2 units a year, doubling in less than three years, and patient having the metabolic syndrome, defined as men overweight, diabetic, with elevated fat and cholesterol reading.

The "pussy cat" will have a Gleason Grade of 6 or less, have positive biopsies in less than half the number of total needles shot, and the tumour will occupy less than 10% of the sample core.

How safely can this population with low-grade cancer be followed? Currently, active surveillance is strongly promoted for this population. Doing more is considered overtreatment. In Toronto. Lorry Klotz advised this on his patient population, but when he eventually took some of these patients to surgery, because they advanced or demanded it, twenty-five per cent had positive margins and eight per cent had positive lymph nodes. Certainly, for this group, active surveillance failed them, when earlier surgery could have cured them.

Perhaps Magnetic Resonance Imaging (MRI) will resolve this problem. MRI can indicate the size of the area of suspicion, and tumours of less than 3 ml are considered insignificant, those 4 to 5 ml intermediate in significance, and those over 5 ml significant. Should all men with a 4-5 ml, Gleason 6 tumour be advised to have active surveillance?

Magnetic Resonance Imaging of the prostate will become more and more popular in the years ahead. Many experts feel that this test should precede ultrasound-guided biopsies, which may be rendered unnecessary in many instances. Furthermore, when the biopsy is done before the magnetic scan, it distorts the images, making the interpretation more difficult. But, an MRI on every man with an elevated PSA is very costly and not possible with present facilities. (In a private lab the test currently costs $850 in Montreal.) Furthermore, interpretation of the scans requires trained expertise. It will be interesting to see how we, as a society, resolve these issues.

HORMONE TREATMENT

The objective of hormone treatment is to get the patient's testosterone level down to zero – or close to zero – so that it will not help the prostate tumour to grow. (Prostate cancer is thought to be nourished by testosterone, remember.) It is used mostly when a patient has cancer that has already spread by the time his diagnosis is made.

Androgen Deprivation Therapy (ADT) or hormone treatment consists of:

- Orchiectomy, the surgical removal of the testicles;
- Anti-fungal pill called Nizoral (ketoconazole);
- Injections of drugs known as LHRH agonist that block testosterone production;

- The agonist works by instructing the brain to stop producing a hormone that stimulates the testicles to make testosterone. Initially, there is more testosterone production, which is known as the flare;
- Injections of a drug known as LHRH antagonist, Firmagon (degarelix), which stops testosterone from being produced without the initial testosterone elevation;
- Anti-androgen pills that block testosterone from entering prostate cells as well as preventing it from being made by the adrenal gland;
- A drug that blocks synthesis of testosterone by the adrenal gland and even, perhaps, by prostate cancer cells – Zytiga (abiraterone);
- A drug that blocks the transport of testosterone from outside the cell nucleus to the inside thus inhibiting tumour cell survival – Enzalutamide (Xtandi).

Calling hormone treatment "palliative" treatment, as is often the case, is unduly pessimistic. Almost all – perhaps ninety-five percent – of men initially respond to it quite positively. These range from up to four percent who are actually cured by it, or who show no evidence of further disease while having it, to nearly fifty percent who stay controlled beyond two years.

One of these men, I recall, was a healthy, fifty-two-year-old electronic technician who was surprised to learn that his PSA reading was an astounding 83! That's when he first came to see me. My investigations revealed that he had an advanced tumour. An ultrasound-guided biopsy revealed a Gleason Grade 8 in all six needles (six being the usual number used at that time), and a bone scan showed metastatic disease in his low back bones. In effect, this man had M1b or D2 disease.

Hormone therapy was started immediately and, within only a

month or so, the patient's PSA had dropped to 0.24. Today, more than eight years after consulting me, with panic in his face, he has no detectable disease.

He is one of the lucky ones. While, as I have said, half of the patients who have hormone treatment are definitely helped by it, the other fifty percent do not fare as well on it at all. They demonstrate slow, but progressive, disease within two years of starting the treatment, and, unfortunately, die. I should be quick to add, however, that these men are most often elderly, and much older than was our electronic technician.

Alas, the best hormone treatment in the world is by no means the panacea. We know it can help an advanced cancer, but there is often nothing that can be done to alleviate other, unrelated health problems that afflict some elderly men. Such was the case of yet another retired physician who sought me out. He had a Gleason Grade 9 cancer with a PSA reading of 21.7. He typified the kind of patient who would naturally profit from hormone treatment, except that after starting it he was diagnosed with progressive kidney failure.

I carried out an orchiectomy on him when his PSA rose to 36, and he quickly found himself in remission with a PSA of zero. Since then, however, his kidneys have deteriorated; because he is now seventy-eight years old, all we can do is monitor him carefully with that "watchful waiting," and keep him comfortable

The main advantage of the orchiectomy is that it can reduce a man's testosterone level to what we call "a castrate level" within a matter of hours, while pills and injections may take days, even weeks.

There are two ways to perform an orchiectomy. One method is called the bilateral orchiectomy, which means that the entire testicles are removed, and the other is known as a subcapsular orchiectomy. In this, the surgeon takes out only the interiors of the testicles, leaving the outer shells. This method is equally as effective as the bilateral one, and in no way compromises treatment because there are no testosterone-producing cells in the outer shells of the testicles.

The subcapsular removal of the testicles does, however, have the advantage of maintaining a semblance of normal male anatomy – for psychological reasons, if nothing else. If I had to have an orchiectomy to control prostate cancer, I would insist upon a carefully done subcapsular procedure because this operation is less morbid and has fewer complications.

You may ask another of my patients about this – a sixty-two-year-old father of two pre-teen children whose advanced prostate cancer had already spread into his bones when he arrived at my office. His biopsy showed a Gleason 9 cancer.

I performed a subcapsular orchiectomy on him and installed a testicular prostheses in his scrotum because he said he wanted to have a "normal" body so he would not feel awkward when he went to the local pool with his children.

He also opted for anti-androgens. Fourteen years after surgery, his PSA was zero, and he was fine except for the constant fear that his cancer may return.

The next quickest way to lower the testosterone level, after the orchiectomy, is by using the anti-fungal drug, Nizoral (ketoconazole). The 200-mg tablet has to be administered in a dosage of one 200-mg tablet three times per day. With this, castrate levels of testosterone are achieved within twenty-four hours but are maintained only while taking this drug. The negatives of this treatment are nausea, intolerance, and loss of effect after a few months.

The least expensive way to lower the testosterone to castrate level is with the female hormone pill, DES (stilboestrol). 3 mg per day is the standard dose to achieve this effect in two weeks, but 1 mg may suffice. This treatment has fallen into disfavour, however, because of cardiovascular complications that have been assigned to it. DES causes fluid retention and increases the risk of heart attacks, and inflamed blood clots in the legs (thrombophlebitis), which may lead to a potentially fatal blood clot in the lungs (pulmonary embolism).

Whenever I prescribe DES, I always tell the patient to take the common Aspirin with it to lessen these risks. An anticoagulant like Coumadin (warfarin), may produce even more successful results in preventing cardiovascular complications.

Another useful hormone-treatment drug which can also be used to drop testosterone levels is a progesterone-like hormone pill called Androcur (cyproterone acetate). This has become very popular in Canada and in Europe, although it is not available in the U.S. It has the dual effect of suppressing testosterone production from the testicles as well as blocking its entry into prostate cells. Unlike most hormonal medications, it does not cause hot flashes as a frequent side effect.

Critics of this particular drug argue that it is less likely to achieve castrate levels of testosterone than other medications or orchiectomy, that a patient's PSA may not fall as low as it might, and that there are increased risks of blood clots, as well as extreme muscle fatigue. Many patients have responded well to it, though, especially when it has been taken with small doses of DES (0.1 mg a day). Furthermore, when patients are faced with surgical castration because of their cancer, they nearly always prefer to take a simple pill, and, when they do well on it, are reluctant to try anything else.

The most popular, yet the most expensive treatment for achieving "medical castration," is the combination of oral anti-androgens and drugs (LHRH agonists) that are injected into the fat beneath the skin or into the muscle. By this method, castrate levels of testosterone are achieved in between two and three weeks with only one injection. Thereafter, injections might be given every month,

141

every two months, every three months, or every four months, depending on the particular drug used.

A number of pharmaceutical firms compete for this market. Abbott makes Lupron (leuprolide) which comes as a 7.5 mg monthly intramuscular dose, or as a 22.5 mg intramuscular dose every three months or 30 mg every 4 m; Sanofi-Aventis makes the same product, which they call Eligard (leuprolide) in similar formulation as well as a six-month formulation; Astra-Zeneca makes Zoladex (goserelin), which comes as a monthly subcutaneous injection of 3.6 mg, or as a 10.8-mg dosage to be injected every three months. The popularity of this drug is due, in part, to its clever delivery package. No mixing is required, the drug is injected under the skin of the abdomen, and the needle retracts automatically into its container. Aventis makes Suprefact (buserelin), which comes in formulations that lasts three to six months. Paladin makes Trelstar (triptorelin), which comes as a quarterly injections, priced competitively.

These drugs work by stopping testosterone production in the testicles after first making them over-produce it – in effect stimulating so much of the hormone production that all further synthesis of it is eliminated by virtue of exhaustion. This initial stimulation of testosterone output – known as the "flare" – might be considered harmful to a patient with prostate cancer because, by creating a healthy flow of it, the growth of his tumour might be stimulated.

The "flare," meanwhile, can be suppressed by treating the patient with one of several oral anti-androgen preparations for a couple of weeks before administering the first injection. These drugs successfully block testosterone from entering the cancerous prostate cell just as water may be blocked from penetrating a garden lawn by spreading a tarpaulin over it.

The anti-androgens come in two types: steroidal or non-steroidal. Those that are steroidal, Androcur (cyproterone acetate) and Megace (megestrol acetate), have both a good and a bad side. On the one hand, they have a cholesterol-like formulation that is associated with phlebitis. On the other hand, they prevent hot flashes.

The non-steroidal anti-androgens, however, are the ones most popular today, and therefore the most commonly prescribed. One of these, Euflex (flutamide), is a pill that must be taken three times a day and is fairly innocuous, causing rare intestinal upsets and – even rarer – liver damage as side effects. Another medication, Anandron (nilutamide), is taken three times daily in 100-mg tablets. Unlike Euflex it has no intestinal side effects at all, although some patients complain that it makes them extra sensitive to sunlight.

Many years ago I was invited, by the drug company Hoechst-Roussel, to a think-tank session designed to find out why its Anandron was not competing well against Schering's Euflex, and how it could improve its sales of this very useful drug. It is always difficult, after all, for a company to break into the market with a new drug when an earlier one has become so well established, and when there is no real difference in clinical effectiveness between the two.

The difference here, I'd decided, was solely in each drug's side effects, and with this in mind I suggested that Hoechst-Roussel might provide urologists with free sunglasses to give to those patients who were about to take Anandron. The idea might serve as a reminder to the urologist to tell the patient that wearing sunglasses – for free, no less! – might be better than suffering cramps and diarrhoea and risking that liver damage.

The company did not adopt my idea because its management felt it would emphasize the drug's negative aspects far too much. Later on, without improved sales, those same company officials admitted that I might have had a point.

The third and latest available non-steroidal anti-androgen is Casodex (bicalutamide) made by Astra-Zeneca. This has the advantage of having to be taken only once day, a 50-mg tablet at a time, and its side effects are almost non-existent.

The combined use of anti-androgens and the injections should maximize the blockage of male hormone effects, and this "total" or "maximum" androgen blockade should improve the prognosis for patients with advanced prostate cancers.

Many studies have been done on the value of using a combination of these pills and injections to block testosterone, but they are divided on the success rates. In a large-scale study done in the U.S., both a rising PSA and the time-to-death rate was unaltered by adding anti-androgens to surgical castration. It is still not clear whether the addition of anti-androgen pills to injection treatment, that is, the LHRH agonists, prolongs the life of a man suffering from advanced prostate cancer.

More certain is that while medical castration can be reversed, surgical castration cannot. Stopping the injections will eventually restore the testosterone level, although it may take between three and six months, or even longer, for the hot flashes to disappear and the libido to return.

Investigators in Vancouver have proposed cyclical hormonal therapy, not only for psychological reasons but because the animal experiments they had done suggested that the periodic restoration of a normal testosterone environment kept cancer cells from developing hormone independence.

Put another way: when testosterone is eliminated from the body, certain cancer cells that do not depend on it for survival, and are normally held it check by it, are allowed to flourish. Practically, then, routine hormonal treatment is stopped when a patient's PSA reaches the nadir, or lowest level, so as to allow the testosterone to reappear. The treatment is re-started when the PSA rises again. One such regime starts treatment when the PSA reaches 10 and stops it when the PSA drops to 4.

This cyclical treatment has yet to be fully time-tested, but if it is more effective than, or even as good as, continuous treatment, it would represent a strong argument in favour of medical castration over surgical castration. It should also be remembered that by allowing his testosterone to reach a "normal" level, a patient's psychological health is restored.

Historically, there has been no difference in prostate cancer survival rates, whether testosterone levels have been lowered by surgical orchiectomy or controlled by estrogens and progestational agents, or by injections. Nor have there been advantages in adding one modality of treatment to another – giving injections to a man who has had a surgical orchiectomy, for example, or estrogens to another who has been getting injections.

What little differences that are evident have been seen in psychological effects on patients, medical costs to governments in those countries where there is socialized medicine, and in a medication's side effects.

Still another way to achieve castrate levels of testosterone is by using a drug that blocks testosterone production without first stimulating it. This is the rationale behind an LHRH antagonist. Ferring Pharmaceuticals has produced a drug called Firmagon (degarelix), which does exactly that. The drug must be injected under the skin monthly, has some local irritation associated with it, but there is an immediate drop of testosterone to castrate level in three days! It has only recently reached the market, so its effectiveness has yet to be fully established. Early results suggest it is as good as or superior to the LHRH agonists. It is attractive because it eliminates the need to take anti-androgen pills before the injections, but injections must be administered monthly.

I have prescribed Firmagon to newly-diagnosed men who might best be treated with hormone therapy as a prelude to radiotherapy or as the sole treatment. The 120-mg dosage is injected under the skin of the abdomen twice, that is 240 mg is administered. This drops the testosterone to castrate level in 72 hours with no need for the anti-androgen drugs, like Casodex (bicalutimide). To keep the testosterone at castrate level, the drug must be administered monthly. Because there is more irritation at the injection site, I often switch over to the LHRH agonists (like Zoladex, Lupron or Trelstar) after the initial one-month treatment with Firmagon.

Sometimes prostate cancer is controlled by hormone treatment, but the plumbing is not. This was the case with an eighty-two-year-old artist whose biopsy confirmed a Gleason Grade 8 cancer. His PSA score was 25. Hormone treatment was started right away, but three months later the patient could not urinate, and I had to perform a TURP on him.

The tissue removed during his surgery showed the same Gleason Grade score of 8, but his PSA had fallen to almost zero. It was still at this level five years later when the man died of other causes.

Why does one patient with advanced prostate cancer stay under the control of hormones for years, even decades, while another with a similar cancer succumbs to it in a matter of months? At this point nobody knows. It is a subject of intensive research. Overall, almost every man responds to the hormonal treatment, but half will stop responding after two years.

When a patient *does* escape the help of hormones, further treatment depends upon his overall health. If he is bedridden and in severe pain, analgesics and cortisone preparations, along with a drug called Mitoxantrone, given in doses of between 12 and 14 mg per square metre of body surface every three weeks, are all that would be prescribed for him. Mitoxantrone has been demonstrated to help alleviate pain, and, although no reported cures have been ascribed to it, it nonetheless contributes to the lengthening of lives.

By the way, a patient's body surface area for medical purposes is calculated on a graph. A line that connects his weight and height intersects a third vertical line which denotes this surface in square metres. This is used a lot in clinical medicine.

In recent years, drug regimes have been introduced that add, on average, four extra months of survival. One such regime consists of Docetaxol administered intravenously every three weeks along with a cortisone drug by mouth. The latest in this family of drugs is called Cabazitaxel, with a promise of even better results.

Another treatment uses the patient's white blood cells (monocytes), exposed to an enzyme specific to the prostate called acid phosphatase, grown in tissue culture outside the body and reinfused into the patient. This is Dendreon's Provenge (sipuleucel-T), which has been shown to prolong life but costs close to $100,000 per case. Many other drugs are making inroads, such as Zytiga (abiraterone), which targets testosterone made not only by the testicles and the adrenal gland but those made by prostate cancer cells. With this drug, testosterone is dropped to levels not achieved by other methods.

On the horizon are drugs that interfere with testosterone receptors on the surface of cancer cells so that testosterone cannot be utilized. This is enzalutamide, a drug made by Astellas, a Japanese company. Another yet-to-be approved drug is made by a Norwegian firm, Algeta. Their drug, called alpharadin, targets prostate cancer in the bone. In principle, radium substitutes for the calcium, with its bone lethal effect.

RADIOTHERAPY AND BRACHYTHERAPY

Radiotherapy is most effective when it follows a short course of hormone therapy. This combination is called neo-adjuvant therapy, and it is becoming the established treatment when surgery is not the best option.

When it is given first, hormone therapy shrinks the gland and provides a smaller target for radiotherapy later, thus reducing the chances of radioactive spillover into adjacent sites and the side effects this may create. Furthermore, as recent reports have indicated, the combination of radio and hormone therapy improves results.

Three-dimensional conformal radiotherapy is a term used to describe a computer-assisted configuration of the prostate to guide the radiation. The prostate gland is more precisely attacked with this technique, and even larger doses of radiation can also be administered without overflowing into unwanted area.

The total cumulative amount of "rads," or centigrays (cGy), is critical. For prostate cancer, about 6000 to 7000 cGy must be delivered, usually in about thirty-five treatment sessions, each lasting fifteen minutes. Skipping Saturdays and Sundays, the entire treatment thus takes about seven weeks. If there is an interruption in the treatment because of an illness, it is not necessary to restart it; the important factor is the total amount of radiation administered over a given period.

Radiation can also be delivered by radioactive pellets, or seeds, that are placed inside the prostate gland itself. This technique is called brachytherapy. Back in the 1970s, doctors at New York City's Memorial Sloan Kettering Hospital placed seeds of radioactive iodine into a patient's prostate after exposing the gland with a surgical incision below the navel. The results were not impressive, and the procedure was abandoned.

Brachytherapy resurfaced, however, with the development of ultrasound-guided placement of two kinds of pellets – one containing radioactive iodine, the other radioactive palladium. In this procedure, the patient is placed in an exaggerated child-bearing position. An ultrasound probe is inserted into his rectum, and a thick, metal template, with pre-set holes, is placed on the perineum, the space between the scrotum and anus. The holes in the thick template allow a series of needles to be inserted parallel, and evenly.

The radioactive iodine pellets are placed inside the prostate at varying depths to ensure an even distribution of the radiation they will emit. In one technique, the pellets stay in permanently. In another technique, the pellets are on a string and are removed after doctors consider that sufficient radiation has been delivered, usually after a few days or weeks. The more powerful Iridium 192 is used in this way.

Iridium 192 seeds are more powerful than radioactive iodine seeds. Consequently, they are used only when the Gleason Grade is 7 or higher.

In another variation of this technique, brachytherapy is combined with radiotherapy that is beamed externally at the draining lymph nodes. To improve results, external radiation dose can be increased at will while pellets contain a constant dosage that cannot be altered.

Some patients sail through radiotherapy – beams or seeds – with no side effects whatsoever, while others experience extraordinary fatigue, diarrhoea, cramps, and urinary frequency and urgency. These usually start during the second or third week of treatment, peak at five to six weeks, and then subside. Incontinence is hardly ever a consequence, but erectile dysfunction occurs in up to fifty percent of all patients who undergo this treatment, and this can be permanent.

I should also point out that those patients who suffer from erectile dysfunction following radiotherapy do not do so immediately. Rather, the condition is a gradual one that tends to take several years to peak. Up to fifty percent of all patients treated with radiotherapy to the prostate develop erectile dysfunction. How much is due to the radiotherapy and how much to the ravages of time is not clear.

How does radiotherapy work? Commonly, gamma rays are produced by a linear accelerator. Protons, neutrons, and electrons produce what is called particle radiation. All forms of radiation damage chromosomes, curtailing the ability of the radiated cells to reproduce. This is why the treatment is delivered in small doses daily and why the PSA takes so long, months to years, to reach its lowest level. The reading six months after completing treatment is a good predictor of how well the patient will fare.

What of the other side effects?

In one earlier hospital study, twenty-four percent of patients who underwent radiotherapy displayed genito-urinary symptoms, forty-three percent had gastro-intestinal symptoms, and about three percent had to abandon the treatment because these side effects were severe. Unfortunately, adverse side effects can continue to resurface long after the radiotherapy has been concluded.

Another study showed that rectal bleeding occurred in between three and fifteen percent of radiotherapy patients and persisted for more than six months in three percent of these. Pernicious diarrhoea was diagnosed in about two percent, and cystitis with bleeding occurred in between two and ten percent – a condition that lasted for more than six months in three percent of those same patients.

Bladder-neck strictures occurred in a little more than one percent of radiotherapy patients and incontinence in less than one percent, although the risk was higher in those patients who had already had TURPs.

Despite these side effects, about half of all prostate cancer patients who are given radiotherapy are permanently cured by it, whether it is administered with neo-adjuvant hormone therapy or without it. The results are best when the PSA drops more quickly to near zero levels. There is no expectation of a zero count as is expected with radical prostatectomy. The other half of these patients, however, develop a rising PSA after only two years, which means that their cancer, though not necessarily serious, may still be a threat to them.

Three consecutive PSA increases after it has reached its lowest point is considered a treatment failure. In one large study of more than 500 patients, forty percent who had undergone radiotherapy lived more than ten years after completing it.

Unfortunately, we don't have a precise way of determining how effective radiotherapy can be for any one patient, even when the Gleason Grade and the extent of the disease within the biopsy specimens are known. It is like using antibiotics without sensitivity testing; it may or may not work. It is very much hit and miss.

Still, with more experience, and with better localization of the target, side effects of radiotherapy have lessened significantly. Rectal symptoms can occur in 5-30% of patients, but persist in only 10%. Minor urinary symptoms can occur in 50%, but strictures and persistent cystitis occur in only 5%.

LESS-ESTABLISHED CANCER TREATMENTS

It is human nature to speak less glowingly about treatments with which one has had little or no personal experience. I don't do perineal prostatectomies, which entail moving the gland through an incision made between the anus and the scrotum, and I seem to remember more negative remarks made about this procedure than I do positive ones. My feeling about cryoablation (intense freezing), hyperthermia (intense heating), and the use of laser beams or high-intensity focused ultrasound for the treatment of localized prostate cancer may also be prejudiced.

Cryoablation is still being explored as a valid prostate cancer treatment in many centres, including one in London, Ontario, where my colleague and friend Dr. Joe Chin has won a reputation for being an established investigator. I know Dr. Chin as a competent, honest, and humble scholar; he sees a future in cryoablation, and I trust his opinion. I also feel that the success of this may take several more years to win widespread clinical acceptance. By and large, this is because most urologists have always felt that the trans-urethral cooling of the prostate will not attain the required temperature on the outside of the prostate, where the cancer is usually located.

Today, however, this treatment is not done through the urethra. As was pioneered back in the mid-1960s, between three and eight probes are injected into the prostate in the way radioactive pellets are placed through the skin between the scrotum and rectum with ultrasound guidance. Liquid nitrogen is then passed into the probe until "ice balls" are seen on the monitor. A temperature between minus-180 and minus-190 centigrade is achieved, and this can certainly cause cell death.

Furthermore, the difficulty with cryosurgery has always been how to achieve the proper temperature where it will count most without damaging adjacent tissue and organs. For this reason I suspect that it is enjoying only modest results, and with the danger that it may impair the rectum and the bladder.

At the opposite end of the spectrum, hyperthermia uses microwave energy to attain a temperature of about 43 degrees centigrade. Undoubtedly, when this heat is applied, prostate tissue is cooked. But, as hormone therapy is usually used in conjunction with hyperthermia, knowing how much cancer is killed with hyperthermia alone is difficult to ascertain.

In Toronto, Dr. John Trachtenberg, who trained at McGill and who is now enjoying an international reputation as a prostate cancer scientist, has been exploring laser heat, achieving temperatures considerably higher than 53 degrees centigrade, but only on selected patients who have failed hormone therapy. He tells me that he has been impressed with what the laser can do.

Even higher temperatures are achieved with high-intensity focused ultrasound through probes in the rectum or perineum – 100 degrees centigrade. But this is only attained where the beams, fired into the prostate from different angles, converge. Clinical studies are just beginning on this modality of treatment, but, on a theoretical level, it seems promising. HIFU has been widely used in Europe to compete with radical prostatectomy and is presently being explored as a way to treat only that part of the prostate with disease, as suggested by magnetic resonance imaging (MRI). Dr. Frank Bladou and his team are investigating this form of focal therapy in Montreal.

Using laser energy or focused ultrasound to destroy a segment of the prostate housing the most important lesion, rather than the entire prostate, constitutes focal therapy. Arguments advanced in support of this approach are as follows: if the cure rate and survival rate are just as good, it can be achieved without any risk of impotence or incontinence, and the treatment becomes an out-patient procedure. Early data support these claims. Opponents will argue that we have insufficient data to change tactics when current treatments are associated with impressive results in experienced hands; furthermore, prostate cancer is multi-focal in origin, and destroying just the main lesion makes little sense.

Better definition of the disease with MRI (magnetic resonance) will undoubtedly make focal therapy more attractive in the days to come. We shall see.

The search for the *absolute* treatment for prostate cancer continues, meanwhile, and what we know more positively is that when it is diagnosed early, surgery is more effective in dealing with it than anything to date. Studies show that more patients are alive and well fifteen years after a radical prostatectomy than they are with radiotherapy. When radiotherapy is administered with hormonal therapy, however, the results may be the same as surgery.

Some people might look at these results with suspicion, claiming they are askew, that urologists may have operated only on the younger, healthier men, the so-called "good" patients, and referred the older, sicker ones, the "bad" patients, for radiotherapy so as to be able to boast more surgical successes. Both surgical and radio-therapy results, however, are improving all the time. Sometimes the choice for the patient is obvious, as when he is unfit for surgery, elderly, or morbidly obese.

Often, the choice for or against surgery is made after much homework and deliberation. I try to steer my younger patients with early, but aggressive, tumours towards it, but I generally deter men who are over seventy-two years old, and those with extensive local disease, towards radiotherapy. So, while the palliative option is hormone treatment, the curative options are very definitely ra-diotherapy – or surgery.

Protracted hormone therapy in men with more advanced dis-ease is associated with significant bone loss, as is the case in post-menopausal women. This has become a subject of increased interest in recent time. I prepared an opinion paper published in February 2012. Although my essay was meant for doctors, it should be un-derstandable enough for a general readership. As this book is meant for a general readership, you can choose to skip it if you wish.

ESTROGENS IN THE TIME OF BLOOD-THINNERS

In the heyday of their use, estrogens were immensely popular in the treatment of men with advanced prostate cancer and older women who cherished a younger body. Estrogen combined with proges-terone constituted Hormone Replacement Therapy (HRT) and was considered beneficial, as well, for the cardiovascular system, bone health, and emotional well-being. For both these conditions the use of estrogens has fallen into disfavour: in the case of prostate cancer because of complicating cardiac deaths, and in replacement therapy because of a concern for possible breast cancer.

This paper attempts to re-examine the use of estrogens in men with prostate cancer whose disease is no longer amenable to curative treatments like ablative surgery or radio-therapy.

It was in the early 1940s that Charles Huggins, a Canadian working in Chicago, first demonstrated the value of Androgen Deprivation Therapy (ADT) long before it was called that. He showed that bilateral orchiectomy, quickly, and estrogen, by mouth, more slowly, over time eliminated testosterone from the body and improved the health and life of men with advanced prostate cancer. This seminal contribution was rightfully recognized and, Huggins (along with Hodges) was awarded the Nobel Prize for Medicine in 1966. (1)

Surgical orchiectomy remains the quickest way (one hour) to achieve castrate level of testosterone, defined as readings under 0.5 ng/mL, although 0.2 ng/mL is being promoted as the new standard. Arguments advanced against surgical castration have been three-fold: firstly, that it is too invasive, secondly, that it is too irreversible, and, thirdly, that it is too devastating to the male psyche. It should be argued, however, that sub-capsular orchiectomy under a local anaesthetic is an out-patient procedure that takes no more than thirty minutes to carry out and is thus minimally invasive. A testicular prosthesis can be inserted at the time if cosmetic results are important to the male psyche. Sub-capsular orchiectomy is as effective as total orchiectomy, as there are no Leydid cells in the capsule of the testicle. Furthermore, if the periodic presence of testosterone is ever proven worthwhile, testosterone can be administered at periodic intervals. Thus, the overwhelming popularity of the LHRH agonists to achieve ADT must be due to the persuasive sales-pitch of the Pharmaceutical firms. After all, surgical orchiectomy costs a fraction of the annual cost of the LHRH agonists.

The LHRH agonists: leuprolide (Lupron, Eligard), goserelin (Zoladex), or triptorelin (Trelstar) do work, achieving castrate levels of testosterone in three weeks. Initially, however, there is a surge of testosterone, called a flare, which can be suppressed with a two week pre-treatment with an anti-androgen, such as bicalutimide (Casodex) 50 mg po administered daily. There is little evidence to support the superiority of one LHRH agonist over another. Some men may prefer subcutaneous injections over intramuscular, or treatments every four to six months, over every one to three months. The recent introduction of a LHRH antagonist, degarelix (Firmagon), which achieves castrate level testosterone in three days with no need for priming with anti-androgens, will compete for this market although monthly subcutaneous injections are necessary. (2)

Estrogen, which antedated the use of the LHRH agonists, achieves castrate level of testosterone in two weeks. The fluid retention, increased risks of phlebitis, and deaths from pulmonary embolism occurred with higher doses of estrogens, 3-5 mg, than may be necessary, 1-3 mg (3). The Veterans Administration Study revealed the effectiveness of diethylstilbestrol (DES) in treating prostate cancer, but the cardiovascular side effects (infarcts, cardiovascular accidents, venous thrombosis, and pulmonary embolism) often made the patients in the treatment arm worse off than those who had no treatment at all. The risks were higher with larger doses of DES, like 5 mg, but dosed as low as 1 mg DES cardiovascular complications occurred at increased frequency. (4) DES is no longer available routinely. But estrogen, along with blood thinners, like ASA, clopidogrel (Plavix 75 mg), or warfarin (Coumadin) has never been adequately studied and deserves another study.

Smith, Redman et al studied 21 patients on 1 mg of DES and no blood thinners and found thrombotic events in 1 patient, or 5%. (5) Klotz, McNeil and Fleshner placed 32 patients on 2-3 mg DES along with warfarin 1 mg and found thrombo-embolic events in 28% of the subjects. (6) Jazieh, Munshi et al studied 14 patients on 3 mg DES with warfarin sufficient to achieve an INR of 1.8-2.0 and reported no instance of thrombotic events. (7) Clearly, estrogen with blood-thinners deserves further investigation.

There is, however, an even more compelling reason why estrogens should be re-examined.

The aging male, however defined, loses one per cent of his total bone mass every year, but a male on ADT loses four and a half per cent (8). The rate of bone loss after the first year is less certain, but 50% of men on ADT have osteoporosis after 4 years, and 80% are osteoporotic after 10 years. Osteoporosis is defined by bone density studies where the loss is reported in terms of the amount of deviation from normal, with a test value of minus 2.5 or more constituting osteoporosis.

Weight-bearing exercises and supplemental calcium 1000 mg and vitamin D 800 IU can reverse the bone loss as much as 0.5-2.5% (8). But if the loss is 4.5%, exercise and supplements are not enough.

To date, the answer to this problem lay with the bis-phosphonates, which slow the rate of bone breakdown. The oral form of these products, like alendronate (Fosamax 70 mg/wk) along with Vitamin D and Calcium, has been widely prescribed to post-menopausal women. Curiously, the oral bisphosphonates have not been approved for men on ADT. Intravenous bisphosphonates, such as zoledronic acid (Zometa 4 mg/mo iv) has been shown to treat the osteoporosis, but it is expensive ($600 per month). (9) The drug is covered by the government plan in Quebec, Canada, for example, only with evidence of bone metastases that are progressing.

Intravenous Zometa will be challenged by the subcutaneous denosumab (Xgeva) a mono-clonal antibody that targets a rank ligand protein which is involved in normal bone breakdown. In a double-blind, head-to-head contest, denosumab won in terms of Skeletal Related Events (SRE), defined as fracture, nerve compression, need for surgery, or need for radio-therapy. Priced right, it should do well, but it's likely to be priced in the same range as Zometa. (10)

Might there be a valid less expensive solution? Perhaps!

The hormone that builds bone in men (and women, for that

matter) is estrogen. (8, 11) But men on ADT have an eighty per cent drop in their estrogen level (8). The reason seems obvious. Estrogen is derived from testosterone in the presence of aromatase. In fact, women on an aromatase inhibitor are more likely to have osteoporosis. (12) If testosterone is depressed to minute levels, the estrogen must be lowered as well. A small amount of estrogen, perhaps one mg of estradiol daily, may be all that is necessary to maintain healthy bones.

The active estrogen in the body is estradiol. Conjugated estrogen, like Premarin, or synthetic estrogen, like DES, must be converted into estradiol in order to become active. Estradiol is available in pill form (Estrace), or as a skin patch. Estrace 1 mg, at a cost of twenty-five cents, with blood-thinners of one kind or another at different dosages, deserves to be considered to prevent osteoporosis for men on ADT. Its role in managing prostate cancer, as suggested, deserves a second look. At a time of escalating health care costs, doesn't estrogen, with its dual role, deserve a re-consideration?

A one-year study that looks at bone mineral density (BMD) before and one year after launching ADT with or without estradiol can easily be carried out. The study can determine the relative merit of ASA, clopidogrel, warfarin, or other products to diminish the risk of thrombo-embolism. The merit of estrogen therapy can be ascertained or discredited. After all, it is surprising that despite the positive results with DES, with respect to prostate cancer, reported by Scherr et al in 2001 (12), and equally good results with Premarin reported by Omerantz et al in 2007 (13), this modality of treatment has not gained a foothold in urologic practice.

Readers with a literary bent may recognize that the title of this communication has been adapted from the title of Gabriel Garcia Marquez's classic novel: *Love in the Time of Cholera*. Garcia Marquez's description of obstructive prostate symptoms in the same novel, by the way, is more colourful than anything in the medical literature.

References:

1. Huggins C and Hodges C: Studies on prostate cancer 1.
The effect of castration, of estrogen and of androgen injection on serum phosphatases in metastatic carcinoma of the
prostate. *Cancer Res* 1941: 1:293.

2. Klotz L, Boccon-Gibod L et al: The efficacy and safety of
degarelix: A 12-month, comparative, randomized, open-la-
bel, parallel-group phase 111 study in patients with prostate
cancer. *BJU International* 2008: 102:1531.

3. Byar DP and Corle DK: Hormone therapy for prostate cancer: Results of the Veterans Administration Cooperative Urological Research Group studies. *NCI Monogr* 1988; 7:165.

4. The Veterans' Administration Cooperative Urological
Research Group studies of carcinoma of the prostate: A
review. *Cancer Chemotherapy Rep.* 1975; 59: 225

5. Smith DC, Redman BG et al: A Phase 11 Trial of Oral DES
as a second-line Hormonal Agent in Advanced Prostate
Cancer. *Urology*, 1998;52:257.

6. Klotz L, McNeil I, Fleshner N: A Phase 1-2 trial of diethylstilbestrol plus low dose warfarin in advanced prostate
carcinoma. *Urol* 1999;161:169.

7. Jazieh AR, Munshi NC et al: Clinical efficacy of Diethylstilbestrol treatment in post-orchiectomy progressive
prostate cancer. *Proc AACR* 1994; 35:233.

8. Higano CS: Androgen-deprivation-therapy-induced frac-
tures in men with nonmetastatic prostate cancer: What do we
really know? *Nature Clinical Practice Urology* 2008 vol 5 1:24.

9. Aapro M, Abrahamsson PA, et al: Guidance on the use of
bisphosphonates in solid tumours: Recommendations of an
international expert panel. *Annals of Oncology* 2008; 19:420.

10. Fizazi K. Carducci M et al: Denosumab versus zoledronic

acid for treatment of bone metastases in men with castra-
tion-resistant prostate cancer: a randomized, double-blind
study. *Lancet* 2011; Mar 5;377(9768):813.

11. Vandenput L and Ohlsson C: Estrogens as regulators of bone health in men. *Endocrinology* 2009; 5:437.

12. Mokbel K: The evolving role of aromatase inhibitors in breast cancer. *Int J Clin Oncol* 2002; 7:279

13. Scherr D, Reid Pitts W and Vaughan ED: Diethylstil-boestrol revisited: Androgen deprivation osteoporosis and prostate cancer. *J. Urol* 2002; 167:535.

14. Pomerantz M, Manola J et al. Phase 11 study of low dose and high dose conjugated estrogen for androgen indepen-dent prostate cancer. *J. Urol* 2007; 177:2146.

I have reproduced this essay here for several reasons. Every point I
make in the article is accompanied by supporting references in the
medical literature. Furthermore, colleagues unknown to me read
my effort and offered corrections and revisions which I have incorporated into the final draft. Such is not the case for statements that
appear on the Internet. After all, anyone who can type can enter a
statement on the Internet.

There were a few editorial changes in the paper that appeared
in the journal. By and large the changes did not detract from the
message.

My essay did engender interesting comments from different
quarters. Richard Wasserug, a scientist in Vancouver, has alerted
me to the fact that estrogens taken as a skin patch may not be associated with blood clot problems, and that UK doctors are testing the
relative merits of estrogens over other kinds of hormone therapy.
The last word on estrogens and prostate cancer, in other words, has
yet to be determined.

15

PROSTATE CANCER:
Preparing for Surgery

Once the testing has been completed and the waiting period (lengthy for the physician, interminable for the family) has elapsed, the results are explained to the patient. It is never easy to hear that one has cancer of the prostate; however, this announcement can be mitigated by the fact that the urologist explains that the cancer is localized, surgically accessible, and removable.

The very nature of this disease allows for routine surgical removal of the gland provided that the cancer has not spread beyond the margins of the prostate, and even then, there is sometimes hope in these cases, as European doctors have shown. Not every individual is a candidate for this procedure. It is dependent upon several factors, age being among the more significant.

The very best candidates for a radical prostatectomy are men under sixty-five with no other health problems, or those over this age who have good family medical histories of longevity.

They are most likely to have early confined prostate cancer, staged as a T1C or a T2A.

T1C describes a situation wherein there was nothing suspicious on the rectal examination, but an elevated PSA reading led to a trans-rectal ultrasound and an ultrasound-guided biopsy. T2A disease is one that has demonstrated a suspicious nodule in the prostate on rectal examination, and, while the PSA could be normal, it is more likely to be slightly elevated.

A bone scan on a prospective radical prostatectomy patient will seldom be necessary, because this operation seeks only to treat early disease, not that which has spread. A radical prostatectomy, then, is always done with a complete cancer cure in mind, though, on rare occasions it may be a used to control locally advanced cancer rather than to effect a cure.

Let me introduce the preparation for this operation with a philosophical sidebar. From time to time, fundamental shifts occur in the way medicine is practiced. The introduction of antiseptic measures in hospitals and operating rooms was revolutionary and as much a shift in medicine as the advent of antibiotics. Blood transfusions and anti-coagulants may also qualify as being part of a major shift in the broad scope of medical science. The displacement of long surgical incisions by puncture holes for procedures with scopes and cameras may represent another innovation.

The catchphrases of the day, however, are "evidence-based medicine" and "patient-participation in the decision-making process." This means that when it comes to a serious issue – like prostate cancer – patients are expected to do their homework before deciding on what course of action should be taken so that doctors may not impose one upon them, unsuspectingly.

Computer-literate patients surf the Internet to gather information that will help them make a decision. Curiously, people seem to believe in whatever they read on the Internet, even though there is often no editorial validation in what is permitted there. For this reason, many men who come to me with prostate cancer are ill-informed about what can or should be done for them, or have read about improbable cures. It falls on me to set them straight.

Patients are prepared for a radical prostatectomy much as they are for any other major procedure, but there are considerations peculiar to this operation. Before the surgery is booked, I meet with the patient and his partner to lay out the pros and cons. The pros are usually quite simple. The moment I have removed the prostate gland, in a two to three-hour operation, the cancer is gone. The cons, however, are a little different and must be explained with frankness.

First, while incontinence is no longer an issue in this kind of operation – surgeons have long-since mastered the skill of what we call the "nerve-sparing" radical prostatectomy – there is still a one-percent risk of this (treatable though it is) as well as other nasty side effects, such as scarring at the neck of the bladder that may impede urination later by causing a blockage.

There are also risks of wound infections, lymphoceles, phlebitis, and pneumonia. I cannot remember when I last had a case of wound infection. Certainly, there has not been one in the past ten years, because wound-washing before closing the incision in this kind of operation has made a significant difference, and no resident doctor wants to be the one who is associated with the first case of infection to rear its ugly head in some time.

I have, however, had four cases of lymphoceles. This, a collection of lymphatic fluid in the pelvic region, occurs when the lymphatic channels are not clipped during the surgery or because heparin, a commonly used blood thinner, is used to reduce the risks of blood clots. It is not a serious complication, and most cases resolve themselves spontaneously or are relieved with needle drainage, but it is something well worth avoiding because it can retard recovery.

Phlebitis, which, as we know, is inflammation of the veins, can sometimes cause clots that may migrate to the lungs, causing what we call pulmonary embolisms. While the occurrence of this is quite rare as well, phlebitis itself is common and remains a painful condition for some weeks after the operation. To reduce the risk of this, hospitals issue patients with white, above knee-length support hose, and doctors routinely prescribe 5,000 units of Heparin at the start of surgery.

163

Another side effect is acute anaemia, due to a considerable loss of blood during the surgery. To help deal with this during the operation and afterwards, I discuss both the benefits and the disadvantages of a patient storing some of his own blood so it will be there if he needs it later.

A patient may donate up to three units (three pints) during the four or five weeks prior to his surgery. I do not, however, encourage him to do this because it can weaken him at a time when he needs as much strength as he can muster to withstand such a major surgical assault. In any case, when blood is required, three units is usually not enough.

Instead, I encourage patients to determine if their insurance plans will cover the cost of Eprex (erythropoietin), a genetically engineered hormone that stimulates the production of red blood cells. I have adopted the American urologist Herbert Lepor's scheme. He gave 600 units per kilogram of the patient's weight – by injection – two weeks before surgery, with a further 300 units per kilogram if the haematocrit (the proportion of red cells in the blood) is less than forty-six percent just one week before.

To anticipate the probable removal of one of the two bladder control muscles during surgery, the patient is taught how to do a simple exercise – the Kegel exercise – which is designed to strengthen the muscle that remains. Instructions on just how to do this exercise properly is provided by the nurse on the patient's pre-op visit and reinforced either by myself or a resident whenever the opportunity arises.

The exercise entails contracting the same muscles one would use to stop the urine in mid-stream, once an hour during the waking day. When it is properly achieved, the buttocks are squeezed together, and the rectum is made to contract.

In my early days, I did not insist that patients learn the Kegel before the operation, and it is difficult to learn it immediately af-

164

terwards because it can be painful. Yet it is important. Whenever I tell my students this, I cannot help but recall one patient who was totally incontinent. His idea of the Kegel exercise was to strain to push every drop of urine from his bladder every few minutes. Once he understood he had to pull up exactly the same muscle, he rapidly gained control, and his wetting stopped.

By far the most disturbing and overriding effect of the radical prostatectomy is erectile dysfunction which, in as many as seventy-five percent of cases, is permanent. Many men recover their potency after a few months, while others say it takes up to two years. Still more, however, are unable to regain their potency at all.

It is not always easy for a urologist to tell a once-virile man that his natural sex life may come to an end with his surgery, but doctors the world over are forever mindful of Dr. Walsh's admonition that the sole purpose of a radical prostatectomy is to cure cancer, not to preserve potency.

With at least two thousand radical prostatectomies behind me – and having taught two generations of urology residents how to do them for themselves – I disagree with some of my American colleagues who maintain that the procedure should only be done by a select few. It is, of course, one of the more difficult operations for the trainee to do, and for this reason I always stress that attention to detail goes a long way toward reducing the risks of complications. The result of this is that I honestly believe I am helping a new breed of urologist master this procedure.

I am heartened, too, to know that in many of the operations I have performed, the side effects – permanent or otherwise – have been relatively few indeed.

Walking testimony of this was a slightly overweight business-man of sixty who was healthy despite having had a triple coronary bypass operation two years before he consulted me with prostate problems. He had a PSA reading of 8.8, which led automatically to an ultrasound-guided biopsy. This, in turn, showed a Gleason Grade 6 tumour, which now occupied much of the left side of his prostate.

This man, who had already visited several centres in the U.S. and had read all manner of prostate literature on the Internet, came to see me reluctantly upon the insistence of a friend. He gave me a few minutes to study his documents, and then barked, "Are you the very best surgeon in the world for this operation?"

"As a matter of fact, I am," I replied, "but I expect every other surgeon who does this operation to be able to say the same thing."

"Very clever answer," the businessman replied. "I'll get back to you. I have a young wife, you know, and there are certain expectations."

I did the radical prostatectomy a few weeks later, and, fortunately for me – and for the patient – he is dry (incontinence-free) and potent, and his PSA readings are zero.

Another man was far less suspicious when he came to me with a Gleason Grade 6 cancer that had been found during an ultrasound-guided biopsy. Watchful waiting was suggested by a number of urologists he had consulted, and I agreed with this.

Meanwhile, the man's PSA of 7.2 continued to climb slowly, and as it did, we did another biopsy. Now the Gleason Grade was 8, and I suggested radiotherapy. The patient, however, rejected the idea out of hand, considering himself both young enough and fit enough for a radical prostatectomy.

I was persuaded to carry out this operation two years after having first met this man, and I am happy to report that he is dry, with a PSA of zero, and can function quite well in the bedroom for a seventy-four-year-old man – with Viagra! He has since suggested that I might consider doing radical prostatectomies more often on men of his age.

The suggestion that I may have been the very best surgeon for this operation may seem extraordinarily arrogant, but it is intend-ed to reflect the kind of confidence every surgeon should possess. During a court appearance, the renowned American cardiovascular specialist, Dr. Denton Cooley, once claimed he was the best sur-geon in the world.

"How can you make such a claim?" asked the judge.

"Under oath," Cooley replied.

I would like to have been under oath when I verified that one man actually benefitted from his prostatectomy, if you can believe it! He was diagnosed with early prostate cancer in his native St. Vin-cent, in the West Indies, and sought me out in Canada to perform his operation. The surgery itself and the post-operative course were uneventful. Far more memorable was this patient's remark when he saw me during a subsequent visit to my office.

"What did you do, doc?" he asked. "I mean, my erections are stronger now than they ever were before the operation!"

HOW IS IT DONE?

In the twenty-four hours before his surgery, the patient is prepared for the operating theatre. His pubic hair is removed, and he is pre-pared with a mechanical bowel cleanout, with laxatives and with enemas. This can be done at home on the evening prior to surgery or at the hospital in the hours preceding it.

The anaesthesiologist is the first person to prepare the patient in the operating room. He or she places a small plastic tube through the shaft of a needle between the lumbar-region vertebrae, as is done for a spinal anaesthetic. In reality, however, this is not a "spi-nal" at all. The tube is actually in the space outside the spinal canal; this tubing will be kept in place until a day or two after surgery in case it is needed for the administration of pain medications. The epidural has been largely abandoned because the open procedure has to compete with robotic surgery where it is not used. Patients are discharged after robotic prostatectomy two days later, as a rule, and an epidural tube may increase the hospitalization one extra day. Without the epidural, patients are routinely discharged in forty-eight hours.

An intravenous line will be started in the arm in the operating room, and another needle will be placed in the wrist artery (radial artery) to monitor oxygen levels in the blood during the operation. The patient will be put to sleep with a drug that is fed into the intravenous line and, subsequently, a tube (endotracheal tube) will be slipped down his throat into the trachea, or windpipe, to prevent him from swallowing his tongue. As in the case of a simple retropubic prostatectomy, sometimes done for enlarged prostate, a plastic tube will also, at times, be placed in the jugular. The height of the blood level in this tube monitors the blood volume. Now, the patient is ready for me – the surgeon.

16

PROSTATE CANCER:
The Radical Prostatectomy

A world-renowned surgeon was once invited to dinner at a friend's home. Turkey was served that evening, and the host could not refrain from bragging about his ability with a carving knife.

"Look at that cut!" he said, after every few strokes of the knife. "Not bad, eh? And I'm not even a surgeon!"

The physician patiently waited until the self-serving monologue had been completed and then quietly said, "Not bad at all, Bill. Now put it back together, please."

The silence that filled the room was thunderous.

Most radical prostatectomies done today seek to spare those nerves that are needed to maintain sexual function, a procedure re-introduced by Dr. Walsh at Johns Hopkins in 1982, and since modified in many minor ways. What is known as the "nerve-sparing" prostatectomy is still considered one of the more difficult operations for the urology resident to master.

Urologists whose reputations and notoriety is, in some measure, based on this operation, compound the problem by insisting that patients seek out only those surgeons who have performed it more than a hundred times. What is not divulged is how to produce a surgeon who has done a hundred without the first one hundred. And, if we only permit a training urologist to open and close the abdominal incision required for this operation, rather than do the other work so vital to excise the gland, as some of my American colleagues would have it, how will we train him or her to do the complete operation alone?

This attitude of not allowing residents to do very much in the operating theatre is understandable in a litigious society like the U.S., but I wonder how the next generations of surgeons can ever be developed unless they are given diverse on-the-job experience. Thus, at McGill, a resident who has assisted me in one procedure once – whether it be a radical prostatectomy on the one hand, or a TURP, which is a far smaller operation, on the other – is expected to be able to do it next time around with me as the coach.

I enjoy the challenge of this operation. As I scrub up for it with my assistant, usually a senior resident, we discuss all the details of the patient's history, and, more precisely, the location and extent of his tumour. We do this because we want to know just how complex the operation may turn out to be.

If the patient's PSA is under 10 and his Gleason Grade is 6 or 7 (3 + 4), we know we will be embarking upon a fairly routine radical prostatectomy with almost no complications. If, however, these numbers are higher, we can expect something different.

We will have to anticipate, for example – though we are not always correct – that the cancer may already have spread into the lymph nodes. In any case, a patient who has a Gleason Grade 7 or higher, and a PSA above 10, routinely undergoes what we call a lymph node dissection. This means having to cut out the obturator nodes, which are deep in the pelvis, and send them to the pathologist for a frozen-section examination for cancer before deciding whether or not to proceed with the prostatectomy.

Whatever has to be done, as the anaesthesiology team finishes its preliminary work, my resident positions the patient supine for this operation. It is also important for him to see that the patient lies with the break in the operating table in line with his pubic bone.

This is so that when the table is tented up, the patient will now be lying with this pelvic region elevated.

This exaggerated extension of the abdomen is particularly useful for me when I am operating on those patients who are overweight. This position may later cause some back pain, but that has not been my experience. Nor have I found separating the legs for the operation either necessary or useful.

When this has been done, and when the anaesthesiologist and an assistant are preparing for the next phase of their work, I enter the theatre, adjust the overhead lighting and the height of the operating table, and begin my part of the procedure.

First, I paint and drape the patient, and insert a Foley catheter so his bladder will remain empty throughout the entire operation. Now I make the one and only skin incision – in a straight line from the skin at the level of the pubic bone upwards 8-10 cm.

Beneath the skin there is a lot of fat, and underneath that, a thick, white tendinous layer that covers the mid-line muscles. When this sheath is cauterized open, with an electrical current to minimize bleeding, the mid-line recti muscles can be pulled apart, and held apart by adjustable retractors that are fixed to the operating table.

Having pushed the fat aside, I can see both the artery and the vein that run from the abdomen to the legs. These are not important to the work I will routinely do, except that they define the outer margins of my operating field, while the deflated bladder marks the top, and the pubic bone the bottom. The area in which I actually cut out the prostate gland, however, and rejoin the urethra to the bladder, is about the size of a grapefruit.

If I know that I must remove the obturator nodes for frozen section examination, I do this at this time – and wait for the pathologist's report. Usually, the results are returned from the lab to the theatre within minutes, so there is little or no delay with the procedure.

Once I know that the nodes are cancer-free, I can continue with

171

the operation. If, however, they are positive, I see no great advantage in removing the patient's prostate gland. Often, he and I will have agreed beforehand that if the nodes are only minimally involved, I will proceed with the prostatectomy, but if extensive cancer is found in the nodes I will not remove the prostate but remove his testicles under the same anaesthetic.

If no such agreement had been made, I simply close the incision and the resident and I start thinking about which, of all the alternatives that are available to manage the patient's cancer, we must employ.

When the actual removal of the prostate is in order, the operation to do it is begun carefully. I mop away a collection of fatty tissue from each side of the gland to find a thin, almost transparent, membrane of tissue called the endopelvic fascia. I must then cut into this to feel — with my gloved fingers — the side walls of the gland from the base of the bladder to the beginning of the urethra.

Now I turn my attention to a mass of fat and blood vessels that are on top of the prostate at its junction with the urethra. When most of this has been removed, again by electro-cautery "cooking," I apply downward pressure to the prostate to expose two tendons that run from the pubic bone. These are known as the pubo-prostatic ligaments, and their sole jobs are to keep the gland in position.

Cutting them away to free the prostate is not always easy. Beneath these ligaments, and on either side of them, are huge veins. So, if the ligaments are not carefully snipped, and the veins are incised in error, there can be profuse bleeding.

Once I have cut these ligaments as close as possible to the pubic bone, I can depress the gland toward the rectum even more, this time to expose an area large enough for me to tie off the veins. This is one of the trickiest stages of the entire operation, because an error in the next step means a very bloody case, indeed.

To accomplish it, I slide my finger along the side of the prostate, just beyond the apex, and feel the top of the urethra where it contains the catheter. Sometimes, pulling on the catheter beyond where it exits the body will help me identify the location of the urethra. I then pass a long-beaked, MacDougal forceps just above the urethra from right to left, or from left to right. A strong suture is fed into the bite of the forceps, pulled through the mass of tissue that contains all those blood vessels, to tie them off, tightly. I now anchor this stitch with a bite into the same tissue so that it will not slip off.

When the long-beaked forceps are passed into the same aperture, and a cut is made above it, the prostate will have been freed from the large veins in front of it. The junction of the prostate and the urethra can now be cleanly dissected – in a bloodless field. For the moment, however, I am still preparing the way.

I now lift the urethra with the forceps, like picking up a strand of spaghetti – although macaroni might to closer to the actual size – with tongs, so I can get an instrument around it. Because there used to be no adequate tool for this intricate manoeuvre, I had to make one for myself. I went to the hospital machine shop with a pair of tongs that we typically use to hold tissue without damaging it (a Babcock clamp), and filed off a segment of the tip so that it now resembled a carpenter's pincers. I ensured, however, that the bowed tips of these "pincers" were blunt, so that when I used them to lift up the urethra (macaroni), they did the job without bruising it.

Back to the operation: I slip an extra-curved forceps, that is, a Mixter forceps whose tips have been changed from an L to an U under heat, underneath the altered Babcock forceps, as they hold up the urethra, staying very close to it. This is so I will not damage those nerves that are responsible for the patient's erection. A small tape, the kind used to tie off the umbilical cord in the newborn, is then fed into the forceps and passed under the urethra so I can lift it sufficiently to be able to cut it open on its anterior surface close to the prostate – without damaging the sphincter or the valve that prevents the urine from leaking, which lie just beyond.

I can now see the catheter where the urethra has been opened. I pinch it with a pointed forceps called the Schnitz and pull the catheter into the wound. The Foley catheter is then amputated distally where the limb that connects to the balloon joins the catheter. The catheter can now be totally pulled into the wound. At this point I place the two antero-lateral anastomotic stitches inside to outside on the half-cut urethra. I use 0 rather than 00 non-permanent sutures as they are less likely to be broken when tied later on. They will be used to attach to the bladder neck. I then complete the amputation.

With strong upward traction on the catheter that has been amputated distally but which is still running through the prostate into the bladder, I move to the next step. I free the gland from its vascular pedicle on each side, working from the apex of the prostate toward the bladder. This is another tricky part. As I go along the outer side walls of the prostate, there again looms the danger of damaging those same erectile nerves, so I must continue to be cautious.

Here, for the next step of the nerve-sparing radical prostatectomy, I introduce an instrument I have adapted for it. This is used to free the gland from its densely adherent connective tissue and blood vessels, and branches of the same nerves. The dissection must be razor-sharp rather than blunt, and this means I have to cut rather than tease away. When I cut, I must have complete control of the blood vessels before any incision is made.

The instrument I adapted is a curve-shaped set of forceps that carry a silk thread in a V-shaped groove on the outside. I use this instrument, which I had made by a physicist friend (Dr. Morrel Bachynski of M.P B. Industries, a Montreal fibre-optics company), to traverse the outer contour of the gland. The thread is used to tie off all that dense tissue before I make the final cut to release the gland from its moorings just below the bladder. In effect, I am freeing the prostate while preparing to cut it off, and making sure that I don't damage nerves or cause unnecessary bleeding.

AFTER A RADICAL PROSTATECTOMY

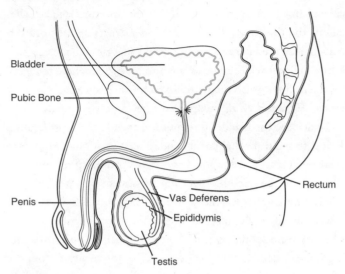

Although this adapted instrument worked very well, it has been replaced by a forceps that cauterizes the bite and delivers a cut in the middle. This has simplified the manoeuvre as well as shortening the time of dissection. Once the gland has been isolated, I can "hinge" it up, or flip it back, and cut into a lining known as Denonvillier's fascia. This exposes both the seminal vesicles and the vas deferens, which carry the spermatozoa from the testicles. In a relatively simple part of the operation, the seminal vesicles are dissected out, and the vas is clipped.

Now the prostate is held only by the bladder neck, and I cut it away little by little, holding it like a dead bloom that is about to be chopped from its stem. The point is, if the preparation is done completely — and meticulously — removing the prostate from the bladder neck is easy.

The gland may now be out, but our next step is to reconstitute that section of the urinary tract. This, too, is a relatively simple job because, if the operation has been done carefully so far, the bladder neck will not have been damaged, and the aperture will, ideally, be about the thickness of my index finger. Years ago, before this "bladder-neck preservation" technique was developed, the aperture was three fingers wide, and this is why a lot of men were rendered incontinent for a much longer period after their surgery than they are today. Thankfully, this worry has been largely eliminated.

The neck of the bladder is rejoined to the urethra neatly, lining to lining, to avoid another possible side effect, a poor urine flow due to scarring. This is accomplished by stitches that bring the lining of the bladder to the outside, "everting the mucosa" as it is called. I use only four stitches for the anastomosis, two of which, remember, were already put in place before the gland was excised. Stitches in the four o'clock and eight o'clock positions, the postero-lateral ones, are now added. All four of these are now ready to join the urethra with the bladder neck. Before finally securing them tightly to make a proper joint, I ask for the operating table to be flattened. This ensures that the stitches will not pull out when they are tied. I then check the quality of the "joint" by irrigating the bladder with saline. The amount of fluid pushed into the bladder should match the amount sucked out.

At this point, I insert a small pipe (a Jackson-Pratt drain) that prevents any urine that may leak from the joint from accumulating around the wound, and we close the incision. The patient is then taken to the Recovery Room for a few hours. After nurses are satisfied that his heart is functioning properly and his blood pressure is adequate, he is wheeled to his room, where he typically begins a two-day recovery period before discharge.

During this time, the drainage tube is taken out, and the patient is kept pain-free, given antibiotics, and subjected to daily blood tests that are designed to measure kidney function and levels of anaemia. As he strengthens, his intravenous and epidural line, if present, are removed, and the nurses encourage him to do breathing exercises to prevent pneumonia and to walk as much as possible to avoid phlebitis.

A few days after going home, the patient's skin clips – I don't use stitches on the skin incision – are removed by a visiting nurse. The Foley catheter, however, remains in place for a full two weeks, until the wound has healed sufficiently well to permit normal urination.

Although any nurse can remove a catheter, I often like to do it myself following this kind of surgery – after using it to fill the patient's bladder. I want to see if he can urinate properly and stop his flow in mid-stream. Even though he may be able to urinate quite well and cease urination on command, he is usually not fully continent right away.

One patient may be "dry" from the beginning while another may not, remaining incontinent for several weeks, if not months. In this case, more Kegel exercises will be needed to help him gain total control, and I want to ensure that he knows this as soon after his radical prostatectomy as possible.

Two months after his prostatectomy, the patient must return to the hospital for a PSA blood test that will tell me if it has been successful. Every six months thereafter, for the rest of his life, he will need another one – this time to tell me if he will require further treatment.

I cannot end this account of what is involved in the nerve-sparing radical prostatectomy without referring again to a patient or two. One came to see me for a routine check-up and, during this brief visit, I detected a little asymmetry and an area of extra firmness in his prostate's left lobe. An ultrasound-guided biopsy later revealed that he had a Gleason Grade 7 cancer.

Because this man was only fifty-two and had a PSA of a mere 2.2, I felt he was an excellent candidate for a radical prostatectomy. In fact, I thought that his good health and relative youth made this the absolute treatment of choice. The patient, however, had other ideas, largely because he wanted as little time off as possible from his work as an electronic company's financial officer. He also thought that, having recently been widowed, he might one day meet another woman and need to re-activate his sex life.

"You realize," I told him, "that if you have radiotherapy first, and it fails, surgery afterwards is not an option. Not at all."

"Oh, why?" the man asked.

"Because radiotherapy turns the surrounding area into concrete," I explained, "and this makes removing the prostate virtually impossible."

"Really?"

"It would be like chipping away at stone to remove your cancer," I said. "Yet, if you had surgery first then needed radiotherapy afterwards, it would be a perfectly good back-up treatment, and one that would be likely to work."

The outcome of our discussions was that the patient would seek other opinions, which I encouraged.

First, he went to Boston, where conformal radiotherapy was advised by a radiotherapist, and where surgery was suggested by a surgeon. He finally decided on brachytherapy as the treatment least likely to interfere with his business commitments, and one that had a good chance of preserving his potency.

This took him to Seattle where the radioactive iodine was placed by my friend, Dr. Haakon Radge, one of the pioneers in this field, and within only a matter of days, the patient was back at work and happy with his choice. I fear, however, that it is too early for us to know what the final outcome will be. More certain is that he must be carefully monitored for as long as he is alive.

Contrast him, if you will, with a colleague physician – coincidentally also fifty-two – who came to see me for his annual prostate examination because his regular urologist was away. This man had a long history of chronic prostatitis, which acted up from time to time, causing him a lot of discomfort. His PSA had been elevated to between 7.6 and 8.2 for several years, but this had been attributed to his prostatitis.

I recommended an ultrasound and biopsy for peace of mind, if nothing else. To my examining finger, the gland was not suspicious for cancer at all. In the report following an ultrasound-guided biopsy, however, cancer had been detected in three of the six needles. This was a shock not only to the patient, but to me as well.

He, like most of the men who come to see me, took my advice when I suggested surgery. Now, more than twenty years later, his PSA is virtually zero, 0.02 to be exact, his potency is intact, and he is fully continent. Still, like a lot of men who have had radical prostatectomies, and have many years of good living ahead of them, he tells me that he has a "panic attack" whenever it is time for another blood test.

While a lot of my patients react in much the same way, I always feel that it is also part of a urologist's job to remind them that surgery is nearly always a cure for early prostate cancer. Before PSA testing was developed, we had no way of knowing when prostate cancer had occurred or recurred. Now that we have it, we are presented with a double-edged sword – whether to know when cancer lurks, or live blissfully in ignorance of its presence.

I think, if I were still relatively young, I would prefer the devil I know to the devil that is still a stranger to me.

ROBOTIC PROSTATECTOMY

The operation Patrick Walsh championed, the nerve-sparing radical prostatectomy, has been challenged in recent times by a laparoscopic procedure introduced by surgeons from France and by robotic prostatectomy with the four million dollar Da Vinci robot developed in the U.S. The robotic procedure uses techniques developed by the laparoscopic approach and has largely replaced it, as it is easier to learn and to do. The reason is that the surgeon using the robot makes moves that are natural and not counter-intuitive, as is the case with the laparoscopic approach. It is not without reason that the company that makes the Da Vinci robot has called itself Intuitive Technology.

Is robotic prostatectomy a real advance? The data to date indicate no superiority of the robotic operation in terms of cancer cures, continence rate or potency rate. Better results occur in the hands of experienced surgeons. Thus, surgeons who do a lot of the robotic procedures get better results compared to surgeons who do only a few, and better results than surgeons who do only a limited number of the open procedures. The converse is true. Surgeons who do a lot of the open procedures get better results than surgeons who do limited numbers of the robotic procedure.

Arguments put forward in favour of the robotic procedure are as follows: the vision is better, blood loss is less, and hospitalization is shorter. This may be so, but in truth, there is little difference in our centre where both procedures are done. Superior results attributed to the robotic procedure are data provided by the makers of the robots. The company has done a remarkable selling job. In 2009, more than 85% of men who had a radical prostatectomy (85,000 men) had the robotic procedure. My colleagues who do the robotic procedure tell me vision is better at the cost of feel. The robot should develop feel, and surgeons who do it the old-fashioned way should use magnifying loops.

There is, however, a significant difference in the cost of the two procedures. The material cost, exclusive of the capital cost of the robot, is about $2,000 for the robotic operation, and about $200 for the open procedure. If results are better with the robotic procedure, there can be no quarrels. But, if the results are not better, and if the taxpayer and not the patient is footing the difference, there can be legitimate complaints. (In Vancouver, patients are asked to pay $5,000 for the robotic operation, half to help pay for the robot and the other half to help with the extra cost.)

How our society, in general, resolves these issues remains to be seen.

17

PROSTATE CANCER:
Incontinence and Impotence

Incontinence and impotence are without doubt the two most dreaded side effects that may follow treatment for prostate cancer. The effects are both physical and psychological, as many men equate their "manly essence" with the ability to perform more than adequately in sexual situations. Incontinence is difficult, embarrassing, and debilitating, as the patient must adopt a rigorous and complex set of behaviours in order to fully cope with this condition. Even with the best care in the world and with the best surgical hands, men usually suffer either or both of these afflictions, if only temporarily. Nonetheless, they are disconcerting disorders, and they are constantly on the minds of nearly all patients as they begin the long, seemingly endless path to recovery.

When administered alone, hormone treatment, which is usually reserved for men with advanced cancer, does not cause incontinence. Eventually, however, it will cause impotence, but this usually occurs at a time when a man will have lost all desire for sex. The very nature of the treatment, after all – to decrease testosterone levels to as close to zero – inhibits sexual desire in a matter of months.

Radiotherapy carries virtually no risk of incontinence, though there are recorded cases of it, but there is up to a fifty percent chance of impotence. The impotence is not immediate, as in the case of surgery, but can occur months to years later.

A radical prostatectomy carries a one-percent chance of total incontinence and up to a thirty percent chance of mild incontinence. The impotence rate, however, can vary between thirty percent and eighty percent.

As a rule, surgeons report better results about urinary control and erectile dysfunction when they talk directly to patients than do independent investigators when they seek this information independently in questionnaires. I suspect this is because patients are less critical when discussing their post-treatment problems with their urologists than they are when they can hide behind the anonymity of a survey.

At any rate, incontinence and impotence are such psychologically crippling complications of prostate cancer that they must be fully addressed here.

INCONTINENCE

Patients invariably ask, "Can anything be done for my incontinence? After all, it was caused by my surgery. When I've fully recovered from what you did inside me, will my incontinence stop automatically? Will I have to wear a diaper forever, doctor?"

If these questions imply that virtually all men suffer a little incontinence immediately after having undergone a radical prostatectomy, so they should. I must be quick to add, however, that it usually lasts only a matter of days. We call it mild incontinence, and it occurs on coughing, straining, jumping, laughing, or rising from a sitting position.

When the operation is undertaken on a patient who has some degree of prostatic enlargement, the thickened bladder muscle which results from this is much too much for the remaining sphincter to handle. The period of incontinence for such a man can be longer than for one who has not suffered bladder-muscle thickening. Whatever the degree of incontinence, a patient always benefits from those Kegel exercises, because they strengthen his sphincter.

I find, however, that when the demands on a patient are too stringent, he doesn't do his exercises at all. Once-hourly contractions are all I ask him to aim for, and this can be quite effective. Of course, Kegel exercises are much better known to women. The diligent practice of these exercises is routinely advised by gynaecologists to treat and prevent stress incontinence after childbirth. The bonus for "Kegelling," as gynaecologists call it, can actually be an enhanced sex life! That, however, is another matter.

While these exercises are very important for prostate cancer patients, there are medications that can help them, too. Some of these, like Ditropan (oxybutynin) or Detrol (tolterodine), Vesicare (solifenacin), Enablex (darifenacin), Toviaz (fesoterodine), and Myrbetriq (mirabegron) work simply by instructing the nervous system to relax the bladder muscles. Other drugs, such as Urispas (flavoxate) and Valium (diazepam) relax the muscles directly.

I used to prescribe Ditropan in 5-mg tablets, but because this drug causes "dry mouth" I ask patients to start by taking only half a pill a day for several days, and once their bodies are used to it, to increase the dosage to half a pill twice a day, and eventually one pill twice daily. I also advise them to have lemon drops, ice chips, candies, or gum on hand. Even then, the mucous membrane becomes so dry that a lot of patients don't like taking Ditropan. Fortunately, a slow-release version of the drug has been released, with less dryness as a side effect, but recent reports of cognitive dysfunction, that is, loss of mental alertness, with this drug has been a deterrent. I seldom if ever use Ditropan in older men, although a cutaneous form of the drug, rubbed on to skin, called Gelnique, is free of cognitive dysfunction as a side effect. I have prescribed this with success in some patients.

Detrol (tolteridine) is prescribed as a 2-mg tablet twice a day or 4-mg slow release tablet daily. It may not be quite as effective as

Ditropan, but it doesn't dry the mouth as much and is free of affecting mental alertness. Toviaz (fesoterodine) releases the same chemical as Detrol, but does so without requiring a chemical reaction in the liver to do so. The 4 or 8 mg pill appears to achieve worthwhile results in days, not weeks, as is the case with Detrol.

Vesicare (solifenacin) 5- or 10-mg tablet has become a very popular drug to treat the overactive bladder. It may be challenged by Myrbetriq (mevabegron), a 25- or 50-mg tablet associated with virtually no side effects. This drug has been approved in Japan, where it was developed, in the U.S., and now in Canada (2013). Urispas, meanwhile, is no longer available, presumably because of insufficient sales.

Drugs to treat the "overactive bladder" have become exceedingly popular in recent years. The need to urinate often should not be the indication for their use. Frequency may respond to cutting down the intake of fluids, and cutting out coffee and alcohol. Frequency associated with urgency to the point of urgency incontinence merits a trial of medications.

Let me mention here what I tell medical students when I have an opportunity to talk to them about the functioning of the bladder. The bladder muscle is unique and unlike any other muscle in the body. When it is stretched, as when the bladder fills with urine, the muscles relax so that there is no increased pressure or tension in its wall. When it is almost full, sensation is felt and messages are sent to the brain. But it can continue to be stretched. Now, when convenient, the bladder can be willed to contract by messages delivered to the bladder via the parasympathetic nervous system.

The parasympathetic nervous system is part of the "involuntary nervous system." The system, by definition, is outside voluntary control, but, in fact, we do have voluntary control of the involuntary nervous system. Eastern philosophies, like Transcendental Meditation, Zen, even Yoga are simply saying we can control the involuntary nervous system with dedicated meditation and practice. Western teaching resorts more quickly to medications. To some extent, frequency, urgency, and urgency incontinence can be helped by dedicated practice. Medications can be helpful, though.

There are also medications that augment contractions of the sphincter muscle. Ironically, one of them is Sudafed (pseudoephedrine), which we know to have caused a lot of problems for men who have an enlarged prostate, and which has mimicked the symptoms in others. This popular decongestant cold remedy, as well as the anti-depressant Tofranil (imipramine), are the commonly used medications to help incontinence by contracting the sphincter muscle.

I prescribe Sudafed as a 60-mg tablet in the morning, or 25 mg of Tofranil four times a day. Sometimes, I combine Sudafed or Tofranil with Detrol or Vesicare. If the patient's situation is improved by these medications, he is told to continue them for two months and then taper them off. It is usually not necessary to continue them for life.

When incontinence remains a major problem that has not responded to either exercise or medications, I carry out an internal examination with a cystoscope – another cystoscopy. During this I can see if the patient's sphincter is working. To find this out, I ask him to make the sphincter contract. In other words, he must perform a Kegel exercise on the operating table.

With the scope in place, I can see if the sphincter responds – or not. At that point, I want to ascertain if there is any scarring at the joint between the bladder and the urethra. If the sphincter – the "tap muscle" – is undamaged but weak, more Kegel sessions are advised, this time under the supervision of nurses or physiotherapists who use a monitor display to show the patient how well he is using the appropriate muscles. Reward, remember, reinforces effort.

If on cystoscopy the sphincter doesn't work, or if the examination does not render a clear-cut picture, urodynamic tests are done.

In these video urodynamics, the bladder is filled through a catheter with a dye that will show up on X-ray.

If the bladder contracts a number of times with what we call uninhibited contractions as it is being filled, it is deemed to be over-active, in which case the incontinence should eventually be helped by Detrol or similar drugs that have been introduced to treat the unstable bladder. The drug called Vesicare (solifenacine) may be the most popular of the lot, but it will be challenged by Toviaz or Myrbetriq.

On the other hand, a persistent "funnel" appearance at the bladder neck signifies sphincter incompetence or sphincter damage. This diagnosis is reinforced when the patient is asked to "strain down" as if to force a bowel movement. A urine leak with a bladder pressure reading of less than 40 cm indicates a severely damaged sphincter.

Such a patient may have to accept any one of the following:

- A lifetime of adult diapers
- A permanent catheter
- A urine-collection device worn externally
- Injections of an animal protein substance to augment the sphincter
- A penile Cunningham clamp
- The installation of an artificial sphincter

Some patients cope quite well with diapers and the occasional use of a Cunningham clamp. This, a "padded clothespin" device, effectively pinches the shaft of the penis and closes it to shut off the flow. When he feels his bladder is full, the patient releases the clamp and allows the urine to pour out.

Other patients prefer a condom-like drainage device. The tip of the "condom" is connected to an open tube that channels urine into a leg bag. Essentially, the catheter does a similar job, except that it is interior while the condom device is exterior and, therefore, will not expose the patient to as many urinary tract infections.

The injection of materials to augment the sphincter, by increasing resistance to urine that has collected in the bladder is, in concept, rather like adding a new washer to a leaky faucet. Teflon, silicone, and various body fats have all been tried, but with varying degrees of success. Teflon and silicone can migrate to the lungs and cause other problems, while fat cells are too quickly absorbed into the body to do much good.

A protein product called bovine collagen, which is made from cows, has been used successfully. To insert it, a cystoscope is passed, not through the urethra this time, but directly into the bladder through the skin in the lower abdomen. I can actually watch the liquid collagen being injected under the lining around the bladder and can ensure that it reaches the right place and in the right quantity for maximum effectiveness.

The results of this simple procedure have been heartening. Improved urine control has been reported in seventy percent of men who have undergone it. When the same injection is tried through the penis, though, it is much less successful because we can't get the "washer" to sit correctly. Because of the bovine origin of this product, it is no longer available, for it cannot be produced without the small risk of mad cow disease.

When all else has failed, a patient who does not want to wear a catheter or diapers or a clumsy collection device will need to be fitted with an artificial sphincter. This is simple in concept but, I'm afraid to tell you, quite crude in application.

The most common such device used today is called the AMS 800, which is distributed by Pfizer, and which can be likened to a miniature cuff that a nurse wraps around your upper arm when he or she wants to take your blood pressure. This bandage-like device, which measures about two centimetres wide, has three pressure settings – between 50 and 60 cm, between 61 and 70 cm, and between 70 and 80 cm – and can be adjusted according to the need.

Basically, an artificial sphincter is wrapped around the urethra and filled with water instead of air. A squeeze-pump inserted into the scrotum moves this water from one compartment into another. As it does so, it either inflates the cuff, thus compressing the urethra to close it, or it releases that pressure and opens the urethra to allow the urine to flow out.

It is, however, less than perfect because, in ten percent of cases, the pressure required to trap the urine causes the cuff to eat into the urethra. In this event, it must be quickly removed. Sometimes it may be safely re-installed, but on other occasions, if the urethra is too badly damaged, it shouldn't be. If we were to install an artificial sphincter on a scarred, bruised, or torn urethra, we would create a lot of more serious medical problems. Urine might leak from the area of the cuff and break through to the skin at the base of the penis, causing all manner of tissue infections.

What needs to be developed is an artificial sphincter that would work under much lower cuff pressure – a device that would be installed at the base of the bladder and *inside* the urethral wall, not outside. This might simply work by being inflated or expanded to trap the urine and deflated to let it flow again. It would not need to do this by squeezing the urethra and damaging it. In other words, I am suggesting a little contraption that could be made to "block" the urine with the simple squeeze of a pump, then be able to "unblock" it to allow the bladder to empty.

If we cannot develop an internal sphincter to work at lower pressure than the compression device we have now, we should be developing an external device that is less crude than the Cunningham clamp. For example, why can't we make a feather-light clamp that would fit a short length on the shaft of the penis with pressure points that can be moved up and down so that constant pressure will not be applied to a small area for any length of time?

ERECTILE DYSFUNCTION

Impotence after a radical prostatectomy or radiotherapy is a subject of much discussion and controversy in urological circles. The problem is how to interpret statistics. For example, a surgeon who claims that all his patients are fully potent after having performed radical prostatectomies on them cannot possibly be telling the truth. For one thing, the nature of the surgery nearly always impairs erectile nerves. For another, his patients did not belong to a fully potent sector of society in the first place, let alone a sexually active one.

Published statistical evidence – gathered for a study by the famed sexologists William Masters and Virginia Johnson – shows that as many as one third of men over sixty are not sexually active, and that more than half of all men over seventy aren't either. This doesn't mean that these men cannot have sex because they cannot get an erection. It does, however, suggest that at the time of their treatment, and the follow-up to it, their erectile ability was not uppermost in their minds. Consequently, they could not provide valuable input to any kind of study on impotence.

Actually, assessments of potency before or after prostate cancer treatment are seldom made, or, if they are, they are not made precisely. This, of course, may be because sexual function seems inconsequential at a time when cancer is the major concern. So, if a man has a weak erection prior to surgery, and no erection after it, he might want to blame his surgeon – rather than the ravages of time.

Nevertheless, erectile difficulties are intimately associated with radiotherapy and radical prostate surgery.

The fifty percent of patents who are *not* rendered impotent after radiotherapy will report penises that are shorter and thinner, but say there is no change in their libido or their sexual enjoyment. Unfortunately, prolonged radiotherapy quite often injures blood vessels, and this is doubtless why the penis may shrink by two or three centimetres.

Unfortunately, surgery can also shrink a penis and render a patient totally impotent, even when a nerve-sparing procedure has been meticulously followed. (Good erections are much more likely to be preserved in younger men than they are in older ones.) It is not clear whether a total loss of potency is due to inadvertent injury to the neurovascular bundles, those nerves that are found each side of the prostate gland, or because of other factors. More certain is the fact that most surgeons will admit to not really knowing if they have damaged the erectile nerves or not.

This explains why I tell each prostatectomy patient, after he has been returned to the ward, "Your operation went well, and you should have no problem with urine control. I'm not sure about the erection, though. We'll have to wait and see."

THE POWER OF VIAGRA

When the restoration of erection is important to a patient, a number of therapeutic measures can be considered for him. For most men, Viagra (sildenafil) will be the first and simplest thing to try. There is no question that Viagra has caused a sensation around the world, and millions of men have tried it. The stampede to the corner drug store after its release in the United States in March 1998 has been unmatched by any other medication.

This wonderful drug, manufactured by Pfizer, works best on patients who are not totally impotent, but is nonetheless worth giving to those who are. In other words, it is most effective on pa

191

tients who at least have a semblance of penile engorgement.

Even older men are aided by Viagra. One of these was ninety years old, if you can believe it, and had been a visitor to my office for some twenty-five years. Many of his friends had passed on, some from prostate cancer, and many others had had TURPs, radical prostatectomies, hormone treatments, radiation treatments, and a combination of them all. My patient was lucky, though. He was still alive.

I suspect he came regularly for his annual prostate examination simply to hear me say, "You have the gland of a twenty-five-year-old!" I might not have been wrong.

One day, as he was about to depart my office, he suddenly stopped in the doorway, jerked back his head, and asked, "Is there any reason why I can't try Viagra, doc?"

I was taken aback at first, but decided to discuss the matter. "You don't take pills for a weak heart," I said. "You don't even take blood pressure pills. You're in excellent health! So there is no reason why you can't try Viagra."

"Really?"

"But as you may know," I continued, "Viagra works only when you're in the mood – and when you have a willing and eager partner."

It transpired that I was making an assumption I had no right to make.

"But, doc," the patient added, "it's my wife who asked me to ask you."

I gave him his prescription and instructed him to take the pill with lots of water, on an empty stomach, one hour before sex.

Patients who suffer erectile dysfunction after prostate cancer treatment may choose to accept their disabilities. Many men I see have done exactly this – often to the relief of their wives, who are glad just to know that their husbands are alive.

Many other patients, though, are not willing to accept a demise in their sex lives, and they equate this to a loss of potency. The two are not the same thing, however, as other patients so often tell me. Men with minimal erections still engage in enjoyable sexual activities, and they tell me exactly what these are. Some of these same men admit that their erectile dysfunctions have somehow brought them closer to their partners, or that their partners have shown unsurpassed compassion and understanding for their problems.

Suffice it to say that when an erection is particularly important to a patient, and he can't get one, I start him on Viagra or another drug in that family, like Cialis or Levitra. It is a first-line treatment. Always, however, there is one proviso: the pill alone is not enough. As I told that ninety-year-old man, atmosphere, mood, and the cooperation of a sex partner is vital for the medication to work.

There are, however, exceptions when it comes to who should or should not take Viagra. Men who are on medications for angina definitely must *not* take it. Patients on heavy doses of anti-hypertensive drugs can take Viagra, but they are often afraid to do so. As an experiment, I ask them to try a 25-mg dose before sex and take note of its effectiveness. Such a small amount of this drug is unlikely to create an erection, but neither is it likely to cause complications. In the event of the latter, I may feel confident in doubling the dose, and this is much more likely to succeed.

When I get requests for Viagra from men who are blue in the face after having walked a mere ten yards, I turn them down, of course.

We must be careful with Viagra — very careful. So, if a well-meaning friend offers you a tablet or two, you should decline to accept it. Almost every one has heard of Viagra-related deaths, and it is a real problem.

So far, about two hundred men around the world may have died in association with the use of Viagra. What is not clear is how many of them died from the drug itself, and how many from the exertion of sexual intercourse. I point out to worried patients that not one fatality occurred during the drug's initial world-wide trials on literally tens of thousands of men, in 1997, and that two hundred deaths do not seem overwhelming when more than a hundred people die annually from herbal preparations.

Nor were there any serious problems encountered when McGill University's Department of Urology tested the drug as part of a widespread study of more than four thousand impotent men. One volunteer, an engineer, complained of bad headaches when he took Viagra. Headaches, facial flashes, and short-lived changes in colour perception (everything looked a little blue, it seemed) were recognized side effects of the medication, too.

"Do you want to come off the trial?" the engineer was asked.

"No way!" he responded.

That was when I became certain a phenomenal product was about to be launched.

When I prescribe Viagra, I usually do so in 100-mg tablets, and then ask the patient to take only half of one tablet an hour or so before sex. Of course, I could prescribe him 50-mg tablets, but, inexplicably, the cost is the same regardless of strength. So, because Viagra is expensive and may continue to be so for some time, I always try to save my patients a few dollars.

Many patients are helped appreciably with the 50-mg dosages, but others find 100-mg tablets considerably more effective.

Two final points about Viagra: first, if it isn't successful on the first attempt, give it a chance. You may need to try it as many as six to eight times to benefit from it.

Second, Viagra has been known to restore "youthful sexuality." So much so, that after having created one erection, it may generate two or three more within a thirty-six hour period – without the need to take another pill. That's three for the price of one!

HOW VIAGRA WAS DEVELOPED

The story of Viagra's rise to fame is worth recalling. Scientists working at Pfizer's British branch were studying a new drug they hoped would lower blood pressure in people suffering from hypertension. Male volunteers who took the medication saw little change in their blood pressures, but were reluctant to return unused pills. They noticed something they hadn't seen for some time – enhanced erections.

What a wonderful side-effect!

The people at Pfizer agreed and began to study the drug for its possible effects on erectile dysfunction.

Was it all serendipitous? Could those volunteers have been wrong?

Actually, once the chemistry of male erection began to be understood, in the early 1990s, it was inevitable that a potency-promoting drug would be developed. The chemical molecule that the body manufactures to produce an erection is nitric oxide (NO). The post-pubertal male releases this from the nerve endings within his penis the moment he acquires those things we come to associate with sexual appetite – sight, thought, and imagination – and when these are enhanced by smell or touch.

Nitric oxide works on an enzyme called guanylate cyclase, which promotes the accumulation of cyclic guanosine monophosphate (cGMP). This compound reduces the amount of calcium inside the muscle cells of blood vessels within the penis, causing them to relax. The sponge-like blood vessels engorge with blood and then work like a flap valve closing the exit door. The enclosed chamber fills to capacity, and the turgor, or rigidity, constitutes what we know as the erection.

After some time, the body releases another chemical product, called phosphodiesterase, which breaks down the cGMP, reversing the process. The erection disappears.

Viagra works not by stimulating the erection, but by inactivating the chemical – phosphodiesterase that brings an erection to an end. Thus, when the "inactivator" is inactivated, the penis is stimulated to engorge.

Voilà! The magic impotence pill – Viagra!

Phosphodiesterase itself is quite ubiquitous. It is in coffee, for instance. And, within this family of chemical compounds, a minor change in formulation makes one product more specific for one organ over another. Phosphodiesterase-5, for example, is specific to the penis, and Viagra (sildenafil) appears to inactivate this specific enzyme.

Viagra can cross-react with the other enzymes. For example, it can react with the enzyme associated with heart muscles, and this may be why cardiac problems can be caused by it. Further, another form of this enzyme is found in the retina, which can account for occasional complaints of blurred vision or that bluish tint about which men complained during our study at McGill.

Pharmaceutical firms like Pfizer claim it costs them $400 million to bring a new pill to market. For each drug developed, ten thousand may have been proposed. Of these, only between ten and fifteen drugs reach laboratory testing and safety testing. Six of these go for phase-one testing, in which healthy volunteers are used to test both the safety of the drug and its proper dosage. A further four go on to phase-two testing, in which the medication's effectiveness and its side effects are studied.

Finally, one of these proposed medications makes the phase-three study. In this, the drug is tested for possible side effects on thousands of patients, usually world-wide. Based on the success of this, the drug proposal is then submitted for government approval.

The whole process of introducing one new drug takes between nine and sixteen years. Most countries, however, will not accept studies that were done abroad, and repeat them for their own satisfaction. This is why a drug may appear in one country many years before it shows up in another.

Still, the manufacturing cost of the pill is minuscule, so fifteen Canadian dollars for one Viagra pill represents an enormous profit for Pfizer.

By becoming the first-line treatment for erectile dysfunction, Viagra has replaced Yohimbine and Trazodone, the only oral preparations in the past with any kind of positive results. In time, it will be challenged by other pills.

Spontane (apomorphine) is made by TAP Pharmaceuticals. This drug, which is placed under the tongue about a half hour before sex, stimulates dopamine receptors in the brain and works best on psychologically based impotence. Its success rate is just over fifty percent, and its side effects appear to be relatively few. There can be nausea as a side effect, but there are no other significant problems.

By the way, I remember cashing in on a side effect. When I heard that a drug used to help patients with Parkinson's Disease caused unwanted erections, I prescribed it for some of my prostate patients. The results, however, were not dramatic.

Vasomax (phentolamine) is made by Zonagen/Schering-Plough Pharmaceuticals. This is an oral version of a drug that is often used in combination with other preparations as a penile injection to induce an erection. The oral preparation has been hard to produce, and excess amounts are known to decrease blood pressure considerably. Nonetheless, a forty-percent success rate has been reported, and this is quite good.

Other pills similar to Viagra have been developed and compete for the market. They are Cialis (tadalafil), made by Lilly and Levitra (vardenafil), made by Bayer. Both these products come as a 20 mg tablet which is equivalent to 100 mg of Viagra. Levitra may have least side effects and has the best record after radical prostatectomy. Patients have safely taken higher than recommended dose with good results. Cialis is long acting, with effectiveness lasting seventy-two hours. Back pain is its most common side effect, but that is uncommon. A daily 5-mg tablet has also been promoted and approved as a treatment for symptoms of enlarged prostates. The most rigid erection occurs most frequently with Viagra. This family of drugs brings more blood to vital tissue and is not nearly as dangerous as originally anticipated.

These drugs, the phosphodiesterase-5 inhibitors, must not be used with nitroglycerin because the combined effect is more than the sum of the two. This exaggerated drop in the blood pressure with the combined use alarms men into believing that they are not candidates if they are on medications to lower blood pressure. Many men are astounded to hear that the erection enhancing pills actually bring more blood to the heart.

Without doubt, pills to help such disorders as erectile dysfunction is a burgeoning field as medicine shifts its emphasis from diagnosis and treatment of serious maladies to the improvement of lifestyles. Obesity pills, intelligence pills, mood-changing pills, and longevity pills, not to mention herbs and vitamins, will become the order of the day. Pharmaceutical companies will spend millions developing these new preparations, and some of this money will be spent entirely on finding suitably attractive names for them — names that will ensure that they reach those corners of the market for which they are intended.

Viagra, for example, comes from a combination of vigour, the essence of male sexual potency, and Niagara, a name associated with the power of the famous Falls. I have a suggestion for any competing product that may lay claim to promoting more orgasms.

How about Morgasm?

18

ERECTILE DYSFUNCTION:
When Pills like Viagra Don't Work

In our society, as in many, a man's perceived "manliness" is tied up in some measure with the function of his sexual organ. Although this is more a myth than a reality, it is nonetheless a severe blow to any man's ego when that organ ceases to function. The number of charlatans who have made millions on pseudo "cures" for this condition is legend; however, there are a few alternatives to which a man can turn in the event that he is rendered impotent, or unable to achieve or maintain an erection.

The problem is that, good as it is, Viagra and other pills like it, like Cialis or Levitra, don't always work, and the urologist must think what to do next. There are several options:

- A urethral suppository called MUSE
- A penile vacuum pump
- Penile injections
- Penile prostheses.

MUSE

The product popularly known as MUSE is a pellet that is derived from the drug alprostadil. It is deposited into the urethra of the penis in an applicator. The patient voids to lubricate the passage, inserts the applicator, a tiny plastic tube about two centimetres long, and then presses a knob which releases the pellet.

Dosage comes in three strengths – 250 mcg, 500 mcg, and 1,000 mcg. Only the two stronger ones, however, are usually effective.

Once the pellet is in place, the penis is massaged between two hands, and, within twenty minutes, an erection should occur. At least, about sixty percent of patients for whom Viagra has not worked attain an erection with MUSE. The downside is that it is more than double the price of Viagra.

When MUSE fails, a patient can still try other options.

THE VACUUM PUMP

This works according to the laws of physics, so it is not surprising that the device was invented by an auto mechanic and not a doctor. The full shaft of the penis is placed inside a plastic cylinder which has been fitted with tubing so that when the device is held firmly against the body, all remaining air can be sucked out of it.

As the air is withdrawn, equilibrium is sought and blood is pulled into the flaccid penis. When a sufficient erection is achieved, a rubber constriction ring is slipped off the cylinder onto the penis to retain the blood. The vacuum is then released, and the cylinder removed.

Not all patients are comfortable with this device, which has been around for many years. Some men find the vacuuming process too painful, and some find the constriction ring too uncomfortable. Other men, meanwhile, cannot attain sufficient rigidity. On the other hand, many patients are positively delighted with a contraption that does not add a chemical to their bodies.

There are several kinds of vacuum pumps. A cheap one can be bought in a sex shop for less than $100, while a more sophisticated one that is medically approved will cost between $300 and $1,000. The most expensive pumps create a vacuum with battery power, and this might be considered less tiresome at a time when a man's mind should be on other things.

Several patients have made their own erection-giving devices, by adapting the equivalent of a bicycle pumps. The best one of these was made by a man who fashioned a $20 wine bottle pump, which is meant to evacuate the air from an unfinished bottle of wine. All he needed to adapt this was a length of plastic tubing, perhaps ten inches long and three inches in calibre, and some strong glue. It worked.

A word of warning: Do not use the vacuum cleaner. Men who have tried this have stripped the skin off their penises.

PENILE INJECTIONS

Penile injections have become commonplace. Caverject (alprostadil), the same drug used in MUSE, is widely sold in fancy packages in 20-mcg doses.

The same drug, sold under a different name, comprises alprostadil in water, a solution that must be made by a pharmacist. Because it is in liquid form, it also has to be kept refrigerated. Caverject, however, is a combination of alprostadil (in powder form) and saline – and the solution can be mixed by the patient himself at the time of use. It does not therefore require any refrigeration.

When Caverject alone doesn't work satisfactorily, drugs called papaverine and phentolamine are added to make a mix. This combined preparation is widely known as "tri-mix."

Erectile dysfunction clinics across the world have taught countless men how to inject the drugs properly into the body of the penis. It is interesting to note that this entire enterprise was started by one man, Dr. G. S. Brindley of Britain, when he was himself long past middle age. Youth must be served, of course, but I wonder why we so commonly assume that an innovative measure cannot be the brainchild of a man older than forty.

There are side effects that should not be ignored. Priapism is one. This is defined as a painful, unrelenting erection that may last as long as six hours, and which, if left untreated, could lead to permanent penile damage and the inability to have erections in the future. This complication is generally treated urgently, however, by drawing some penile blood with another needle and injecting a vaso-constricting drug, like adrenalin. Of course this should only be done by a physician.

Although penile injections are known to work well, many patients try them then stop using them. This is possibly due to fear of needles and a lack of spontaneity, or a combination of both. Furthermore, the side effects include pain upon injection, scarring of the lining of the erectile tissue, which can lead to penile curvature, and, though quite rare, an escape of the drug into the bloodstream, causing heart problems or lowering of the blood pressure.

PENILE PROSTHESES

Viagra, MUSE, and the penile injections of vaso-active drugs have made the surgical insertion of penile prostheses less common today than they were a decade or two ago. Still, from time to time, when pills (like Viagra, Cialis or Levitra), MUSE, pumps, and injections have failed to help a patient, and he still wishes to enjoy sexual activity, a prosthesis is the only answer.

The next question is: Which prosthesis should be installed?

When I treat an older patient who has suffered prostate cancer, and who wants an uncomplicated prelude to any sexual activity, I usually recommend what we call the malleable prosthesis, rather than the inflatable one.

The inflatable prosthesis has too many moving parts that can go wrong, not to mention a pump that is inserted into the scrotum and a reservoir of saline that is installed in front of the bladder. The malleable prosthesis, on the other hand, is one simple piece of tubing rather like a plumber's snake. It can be made to hinge up and down to assume any given shape, which it can hold.

If this implies that a man who wears a malleable prostheses walks around with a kind of erection, so it should. He can, however, bend his penis up or down to whatever position he wants in order to use it. Also, the "hinged" prosthesis is easy to insert and averts other medical complications.

PENILE PROSTHESES

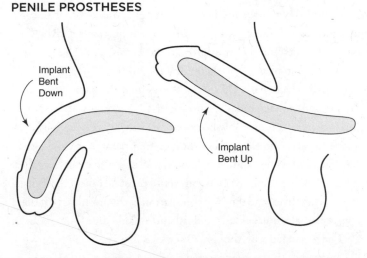

Implant
Bent
Down

Implant
Bent Up

It has been several years since I inserted a penile prosthesis in a prostate cancer patient. A patient's reaction to erectile dysfunction is never predictable, though, and I am forever surprised by it. For example, when a man wants to talk to me about a prosthesis, with his wife in the background, she invariably signals, "Please! Please! Forget it!" Another wife, whose husband has recently battled prostate cancer and is impotent because of it, demands that her husband's sexual functions be fully restored. This is not always possible, but in this, we urologists certainly try.

19

PROSTATE CANCER:
The After-effects

One good thing about my being a urologist, unlike other specialists, such as a cardiologist or a neurosurgeon, is that relatively few of my patients will die from prostate problems, even though they may have been plagued by them for a long time.

It is also true that a US survey shows how the happiest doctors practicing medicine today are urologists! I can only surmise that if this is correct, it is probably because most people are helped by urological interventions, whether they be treatments for an enlarged prostate on the one hand, or help with prostate cancer on the other.

Alas, some patients will have advanced prostate cancer for the balance of their lives, and the only consolation in this for me is that these men are usually quite elderly and will more likely die of other causes.

I have had failures, though. One was a fifty-year-old man who, like so many other patients, came to see me with a suspicious nodule on the left side of his prostate. The biopsy was positive for a Gleason Grade 7 cancer, despite the fact the man's PSA reading was very low – only 1.4.

Within only three weeks of diagnosis, he underwent a routine radical prostatectomy. The pathology on his prostate gland at that time confirmed a Gleason Grade 7 tumour, and one that was well confined. This, and the man's post-operative PSA readings – of virtually zero, 0.03 to be exact – hinted that his problems might have been solved.

They were deceptive, though – especially when the patient

complained of severe lower abdominal pains. Within a year after his surgery, a large lump at the site where his prostate had been was readily palpable to my finger on rectal examination, and from then on his deterioration was swift, despite aggressive radiotherapy, hormone therapy, and chemotherapy. This man died within two years of his radical prostatectomy possibly because the early re-occurrence of his prostate cancer was not readily apparent.

Even in retrospect, I do not know what I and my team could have done differently for this patient. Sometimes, death is just the cruel hand of fate. Nonetheless, I have always felt that all men who have had prostate problems, no matter how mild or severe, should receive urological follow-ups on a regular basis.

Depending on a patient's medical history, follow-ups might include:

- Regular, six-monthly PSA tests;
- Rectal examination;
- Urinalysis;
- Routine history and physical examinations;
- Flow studies and cystoscopies for patients with continuing voiding problems;
- Ultrasound, bone scans, and CT and MRI scans for patients whose PSA readings are rising dramatically.

A PSA blood test remains the best marker not only for helping to diagnose prostate cancer despite the controversy , but for following the progress of a patient after a radical prostatectomy or radiotherapy, too. If his count remains near zero after these treatments, he can be considered cured.

If there are incremental rises in a patient's PSA on each of three six-month tests, a local recurrence of his tumour is suspected. A biopsy can then be tried again, but for a man who has had a prostatectomy it is usually not helpful. There is, after all, no prostate gland to target. For a recurrence following radiotherapy I prescribe hormone treatment, and for a patient who still has cancer after a prostatectomy, a course of radiotherapy targeted to where his prostate once was.

If there is a doubling of the PSA count in six months, I suspect something more serious: a systemic spread of the cancer. In this case I put a patient on cyclical hormonal therapy, which could last indefinitely.

It would be wonderful if we had a scan that could tell us exactly where a tumour reoccurs, but we don't. The next best thing to this is the ProstaScint, a scan test that is meant to tell us where the PSA-secreting cells are, by illuminating them rather as a bone scan does. With this, however, there are too many false positives and false negatives to make it consistently useful. Besides, this test is prohibitively expensive, each test costing about $2,600.

The need for meticulous follow-up is well-illustrated by yet another of my patients, a fifty-nine-year-old accountant. On his first visit to my office, this man only had a mild obstruction of his urine flow. On rectal examination, the left side of his prostate felt firmer than the right. A biopsy of the firm area was done, but it was negative for cancer. One year later, however, a repeat biopsy revealed a Gleason Grade 7 cancer, and, and by this time the man's PSA reading was 10.7.

Soon afterwards, I performed a radical prostatectomy on him, and the pathology report on the prostate I had cut out revealed extensive cancer in the left lobe – a tumour that was approaching, but not invading, the edges of the tissue removed. In other words, this man's cancer was on the verge of escaping from the gland.

Subsequent six-monthly PSA blood test levels were close to zero for four years, but then they started to rise. Within a further four years they had gone from 0.7 to a worrisome 4.6, but the patient had no ill-effects whatsoever. He urinated well and was able to have an erection.

Nonetheless, I decided that his cancer had reoccurred, and I treated him accordingly with hormones – Casodex (bicalutimide), to block testosterone from entering the prostate cells, and Zolodex (goserelin) to stop the testicles from making it. I was then happy to see his PSA fall to 0.2.

When I stopped this treatment, the patient's PSA shot up again, to 1.4. At this point, he and I decided on a bone scan, which was negative. Radiotherapy to the prostate bed was then agreed upon, and after its completion the patient's PSA dropped back to below 1. Today, more than twenty years after his prostatectomy, his PSA is still low and – more important – he is enjoying his life.

This case illustrates several points. It is not unusual for patients who are seemingly cured with zero PSAs to suddenly see their PSA levels rise some years after having had surgery. It is also not unusual for such a patient to respond to hormone therapy or radiotherapy. In fact, we might even ask: would he have been better off without the surgery in the first place? Or, is he better off today because of the surgery? The answer, of course, is that we don't really know because we are not blessed with hindsight.

What we are more sure about is that even though a patient is not cured by surgery – and it is naive to think that everyone will be – the progression of his disease will not necessarily be accelerated. Only on rare occasions do patients in whom cancer cells are left suffer a disturbing progression of their tumours like a fire out of control.

There are two schools of thought about which patients should have radical prostatectomies, and which shouldn't. At the moment, of course, these operations are generally confined to healthy men who, as we have discussed, are under seventy, who have early confined disease, and who have ten good years of life ahead of them.

Some urologists, like Dr. Thomas Stamey, believe that if the prostate is more than forty percent invaded by a tumour, there is no point in removing it because a cure may be impossible. Dr. Alan

Parton reinforces this view with an elaborate table that gives odds for the likelihood of a surgical cure based on different levels of PSA readings combined with different designations of the Gleason Grade.

These doctors feel that by making a man undergo surgery that may not be curative, his woes and general well-being will be compromised as he struggles to recover. It would be better, they say, to supplant surgery with radio or hormone therapy almost immediately after the tumour has been found to be extensive – as a softer way to go.

Other doctors, however – particularly those at the Mayo Clinic, in Rochester, Minnesota – hold an opposite view. They think that denying a patient a prostatectomy because his cancer may be locally extensive, and relying solely on hormone treatment and radiotherapy, is somehow accepting that surgery has no role to play in prolonging life when a tumour may be advanced.

I agree with that. I feel strongly that it is wrong to administer only palliative-type treatment so soon after diagnosis, and that the radical prostatectomy has a role for many cancer patients, regardless of how extensive their tumours may be within the gland. Surgery may not actually rid a man of all of his cancer, of course – something we won't know, even following pathology reports during and after the operation itself – and it may well have spread.

That problem is conceded. Radical surgery will, however, help the patient alleviate any urinary problems he may suffer later because his cancerous prostate may be enlarged. It may even prevent kidney damage should his urine back up, and the severe, unrelenting pain that this incurs.

Not only this, there is a strong psychological yearning in all patients to be completely rid of an organ that is harbouring cancer, especially one – like the prostate – which has such a limited use anyway, and yet is so capable of holding a tumour for such a long time.

Finally on this point, we must remind ourselves once more that while hormone treatment can be given at any time, surgery cannot follow any radiotherapy that may have failed. Radiotherapy can, however – and must – be given when cancer recurs after surgery.

Admittedly, there have been many cases when, on hindsight, a radical prostatectomy may have been unnecessary. Against this, though, there is no defence. When there are overwhelming indications of cancer we have no alternative but to surge ahead. I once treated a man who was seventy when he was diagnosed with an early prostate tumour. I proposed a curative radical prostatectomy. The patient had other ideas; he wanted to delay the procedure until he had completed psychiatric treatment for depression. In the interim he agreed to hormonal treatment – until his psychiatrist persuaded him to go for the surgery.

To my surprise, when the prostate was removed, the pathologist couldn't find any cancer in it. He was stunned, and, fearing a misdiagnosis, promptly rechecked the biopsy I had taken before the operation. Lo and behold, cancer had been there all right, but now it was gone! I suspect that the patient's tumour was among the four percent that are completely eradicated by hormone treatment.

Why do some patients, even those with advanced prostate cancer, stay controlled by hormones for many years, even decades, while other with a similar cancer succumb to it in a matter of months? At this point nobody knows the answer. It is a subject of intensive research.

In general, urologists believe that hormonal therapy almost always works for two years, after which, fifty percent will have rising PSA denoting further disease that is hormone resistant. It should be remembered, though, that the other fifty percent stay controlled.

When patients are no longer helped by hormone therapy, that is, androgen deprivation therapy, further treatment depends upon their overall health. If a man is bedridden and in severe pain, no attempts are made to fight the cancer. From then on, his treatment truly is palliative. Pain control and cortisone preparations, along with a drug called Mitoxantrone (between 12 and 14 mg per square metre of body surface every three weeks), are all that will be prescribed for him. Mitoxantrone has been demonstrated to help alleviate pain, and although no cures can be attributed to it, it may lengthen lives.

PALLIATIVE RADIOTHERAPY

If the pain from prostate cancer in the bones is well localized, spot-radiation to the site is very effective for symptomatic relief. There may be increased pain for two to three days immediately after the radiation – ironically a sign of good results – and then complete relief after one or two weeks. Happily, I can report that palliative radiation controls pain in between eighty and ninety percent of patients.

Radiation that is not for cure, but for the relief of symptoms, has been used as well when a tumour has collapsed a vertebra and the spinal cord or nerve roots are compressed. It is effective, too, when there is urinary bleeding, a blockage in a ureter, or when there is a distressing pain deep in the lower abdomen, at the site of the prostate.

When there is extensive cancer in the backbone, or vertebral body, it can collapse and shorten the bone, and, at the same time, expand one of the cartilaginous discs that lie between the vertebrae. This expansion of the disc places pressure on the spinal cord, causing severe pain that brings on neurological signs or symptoms.

Patients say they feel "electric shocks" in their legs, increased sensations to slight touches, lessened sensations or numbness, or even paralysis. The collapse of the bone and the protrusion of the disc can be diagnosed by a nuclear magnetic scan, or by a CT scan combined with a dye that is injected into the spinal canal in a procedure known as a myelogram.

If such a patient is not already on hormonal therapy, this is started immediately. Because of its fast action, Ketaconozole, an anti-fungal agent, may be the treatment of choice. Then, radio-therapy is begun.

Neuro-surgical intervention (nerve decompression) is considered if the spine is unstable, when there is neurological deterioration while the patient is on radiotherapy, or when he suffers nerve compression to areas that were previously radiated. Often, this kind of surgery, a judgment call, is performed by neurosurgeons or orthopaedic surgeons.

Radiotherapy for nerve compression relieves not only the pain in more than ninety percent of cases, but improves the neurological status in about two thirds of them. The treatment to control bleeding, to open up a blocked ureter, or to provide relief for patients with intractable pelvic distress, is often tried, usually out of desperation, but there are only occasional happy outcomes.

PALLIATIVE PAIN CONTROL

Pain management has become a specialized art. Doctors involved in palliative – often terminal – care provide most of the expertise. They utilize various combinations of drugs starting with Codeine, progressing to Duragesic (fentanyl) or Percocet (oxycodone), and finally graduating to the better known morphine and dilaudid.

Many of these drugs are formulated to be long-acting so that they only need to be taken twice a day. Shorter-acting drugs are used to establish the right dosage. 10 mg of morphine by injection, or 20 to 30 mg by mouth, will control pain for between three and four hours. The equivalent dose for Codeine is 120 mg by injection or 180 to 240 mg by mouth; for Percocet, the equivalent dosage is 15 mg by injection, 10 to 15 mg by mouth; and for Dilaudid, 2 mg by injection or between 20 and 30 mg orally.

Duragesic, which is sold as a skin patch containing fentanyl, comes in four different strengths, and the effects of each patch last three days. Patients are usually started with a 25 mcg/patch which is changed every 72 hours and titrated up as necessary to a maximum 100 mcg/patch.

In addition to pain-controlling medications, bowel softeners such as Colace (docusate), laxatives like Senokot (senna), and anti-nausea preparations like Maxeran (metoclopramide) can be very helpful in making patients more comfortable. Mental agitation, hallucinations, and delusional thoughts that precede death are best treated with 5 mg of Haldol (haloperidol) three times a day.

CHEMOTHERAPY

In recent times, taxol-based chemotherapy, Taxotere, (docetaxel) replaced most other traditional chemotherapy. The oncologists inject Taxotere intravenously, the dosage based on body weight (75 mg/m square IV every three weeks) and administer cortisone (Prednisone) at the same time. Results indicate a definite prolongation of life, but only by three to four months. When Taxotere is not effective, a second line cytotoxic chemotherapy with a drug called cabazitaxel (25 mg/m square IV every three weeks) has proven to have short-term value.

There has also been a startling innovation in hormone therapy as well. Traditional attempts to lower testosterone levels to zero were not always successful, because the adrenal gland and possibly prostate cancer cells themselves may manufacture testosterone. A new drug called Zytiga (abiraterone 1000 mg orally daily along with prednisone 10 mg/day) blocks testosterone produced in this way. The drug is now approved and has changed the course of patients who were progressing on the standard hormone therapy. Another oral drug called Xtandi (enzalutimide) taken at a dosage of 160 mg per day has been introduced even more recently with promising results, as it blocks the normal pathway of testosterone from cell cytoplasm to cell nucleus.

Targeted chemotherapy has also gained popularity. Some, such as Atrasenten, an Abbott drug, has been abandoned, but others, such as alpharadin, developed by the Norwegian firm Algeta, are showing early promise.

EXPERIMENTAL THERAPY

For now, some therapies for prostate problems are far too experimental to be used — even as backups when all other treatments have failed. If they turn out to be worthwhile, however, they may well replace hormone therapy, radiotherapy, even surgery, as the definite treatments.

These new therapies are:

- Angiogenesis inhibitors;
- Gene therapy;
- Immunotherapy.

Angiogenesis inhibitors are pills predicated on the assumption that cancer cells need fresh blood to nourish them; so, if we prevent new blood vessels from forming near a cluster of cancer cells, the tumour will be starved and killed.

This effort, which has progressed from the laboratory to test trials, has been pioneered by Dr. Judah Folkman in Boston. Several products are in phase-three trials and are expected on the market within the next few years.

Gene therapy is also still experimental but equally as promising as the angiogenesis inhibitors. Put simply, the cancerous prostate is injected with a virus for which there exists a specific drug to kill it. The virus thrives and multiplies within the cancer cells, and, after sufficient time, when it has incorporated itself as part of the cancer, it is killed off. In the process, the cancer cells die with it.

In another version, a genetically modified virus is injected into the prostate. This thrives specifically in cancer cells that produce PSA. Eventually, the altered DNA kills those cells by preventing them from multiplying.

In experimental immunotherapy, cancer cells extracted from the patient's prostate are irradiated – by X-rays – so they cannot multiply but remain able to retain their collective ability to mount an immune response. These cells are incubated with the protein-processing cells (called the dendritic cells), which are grown outside the body. Now the cells that have been exposed to the cancer cells are injected back into the patient's bloodstream where, ideally, they mount an immune response. The only drug in current practice is the expensive sipuleucel-T, which I have described earlier.

In summary, angiogenesis inhibitors, gene therapy, and immunotherapy are promising leads in the fight against prostate cancer.

Dr. Simone Chevalier is spearheading a project that was first proposed by my patient, Dr. Ashok Vijh, the research director of the provincial producer of electricity, Hydro-Québec.

"Do you think electric current can be used to treat prostate cancer?" he asked. Documents that indicated that electricity could kill cancer cells existed but none, to date, had been applied to prostate cancer. Nude mice (mice bred so that they had no immune systems) harboring human cancer cells grown under the skin were part of the laboratory scene.

Dr. Chevalier assigned one of her students to explore the possibility of killing these grafts with low current electricity. The success was stunning. A medical student, Bimal Bhindhi, extended the study with a second model that secreted PSA. The results were just as successful.

The project has been moved to a dog model, and Hydro-Quebec is involved in producing the apparatus to generate the appropriate direct current electricity. Time will tell if we are on to anything or not!

THE BOTTOM LINE: A CONSUMER ADVOCATE

Reduce your risks for developing prostate cancer. Take anti-oxidants, like vitamins C and E, selenium, lycopenes, and glutathione. Soy products won't hurt, either. Cut down on animal fats, especially those found in red meat and butter. Exercise and stay mentally upbeat.

Find a kind but competent doctor who will not object to ordering annual PSA tests before each rectal examination. Know your PSA level in numbers and do not accept "It was okay" as a complete answer. Get an MRI if the PSA is above acceptable levels, and if that is read as suspicious, get a trans-rectal ultrasound and biopsy (those ten to twelve needles). Ask for a copy of the biopsy report.

If cancer is found, see how it is rated according to Dr. Partin's table, then:

- Think long and hard before deciding on a radical prostatectomy, conformal radiotherapy, or brachytherapy;
- Ask for hormone treatment before radiotherapy but preferably not before surgery;
- Do not neglect your follow-ups;
- Insist on a PSA reading at least every six months;
- Keep your eyes and ears open for new developments, such as a new targeted therapy, angiogenesis inhibitors, gene therapy, and immunotherapy;
- Be leery of chemotherapy, but welcome mitoxantrone and cortisone if necessary;
- Never think back about any decision you make.

Above all, try to look on the bright side and remember that a cheerful, optimistic patient is more likely to be properly managed in his battle with prostate cancer than a sad and angry one.

A Few Words in Conclusion

After more than a half a century of dealing with prostate problems, I have seen procedures come and go, promising leads fade into obscurity, controversies continue, and exciting advances become part of routine practice.

In chronic bacterial prostatitis, nothing has replaced the seldom-used quantitative urine culture before and after prostate massage in order to establish the diagnosis. I am surprised that examination of the prostatic secretion, by the use of a dip-stick, which I have found so useful in my practice, has not been adopted as part of routine practice. When the dip-stick is positive for nitrites, signifying bacteria, I prescribe twelve weeks of anti-bacterial treatment. In non-bacterial prostatitis, the disabling pain, which is a common feature, responds best to Elavil (amytriptyline), despite the development of newer medications, such as Lyrica (pregabalin) or Elmiron (pentosan polysulfate).

With benign enlargement, different alpha blockers (which relax the muscles that choke the passage) compete for a huge market. Flomax (tamsulosin) is the most popular drug, but Xatral (alfuzosin) might be better for younger men who cherish the forward gush of semen upon ejaculation, while Rapaflo (silodosin) may be the most powerful of the three. Avodart (dutasteride) is newer than Proscar (finasteride), but the difference in their ability to shrink the prostate is indistinguishable. I am not convinced that these drugs promote high grade prostate cancer. At the same time, their ability to reduce the risk of low grade cancer may be of little significance.

If symptoms progress despite the two-pronged medications,

surgery must be considered. When the prostate is measured to be 30 g or thereabouts, laser ablation as by the "Green Light" laser, might be the best treatment; however, if the gland weighs 30 to 70 g, the standard TURP remains the gold standard. A prostate which weighs over 70 g suggests the use of the holmium laser, and when the gland is over 200 g, retropubic prostatectomy could compete effectively with the laser approach.

What about prostate cancer? The recent and emerging campaign against PSA screening and the "overdiagnosis" of prostate cancer is, in my estimation, largely misguided. The need to establish early diagnosis of aggressive prostate cancer is paramount. Why should a curable cancer remain the second or third most common cancer killer? Today, we are critical of overtreatment, as we hear from the men who are suffering the consequences of injudicious overtreatment. Incontinence and impotence are not necessarily the norm, but are always a possibility after surgery. We tend to overlook the consequences of undertreatment, because we cannot hear complaints from men who are no longer alive.

We are in dire need of a new and better diagnostic tumour marker: a chemical released exclusively by cancer cells. It may come in the form of a fusion molecule as some recent studies have demonstrated. Time will tell.

I remain curious about the comeback possibility of estrogen therapy. If it turns out that trans-dermal estrogen eliminates the cardiovascular concerns and corrects osteoporsis, estrogens can become the androgen deprivation therapy of choice.

With what we know today, in 2014, the following is what I consider appropriate management of prostate cancer.

Men should start screening – a PSA blood test and a competent rectal examination – when they are in their forties. If the PSA reading is under 2 and the rectal examination is not suspicious; that is, there is no asymmetry in the gland, and no hard nodules, he need not come back for three-to-five years. If the initial PSA is over 3, a trans-rectal ultrasound and ultrasound-guided biopsy consisting of 10-12 cores should be done If the biopsy is negative for cancer, the blood test and rectal exam should be repeated every two years, or every year if the particular patient feels more reassured by so do-ing. A PSA which climbs more than 0.75 units in one year would demand a magnetic scan of the prostate (MRI) and targeted biopsy should be carried out on areas of suspicion.

Patients diagnosed with a Gleason 6 cancer in three cores or less, with less than 10% of the core involved should be monitored with active surveillance, that is, PSA every six months and biopsy every year. Should there be progression, I would advise curative treatment.

Patients diagnosed with Gleason 7 or higher (8-10) cancer, with no evidence of metastatic disease should be offered curative treat-ment. Curative treatment should be a surgery if the patient is fit, and radio-therapy if there are reasons why surgery is inappropriate; age or a heart condition would be two such indicators.

Should the patient fail surgery as signified by a PSA count over 0.2, he should be offered radio-therapy to the prostate bed, with expectations of a potential lifetime control of disease. Should there be evidence of further disease, however, as indicated by three se-quential increases in PSA readings six months apart, hormone therapy or androgen deprivation therapy (ADT) is initiated. The success of ADT will be monitored with regular PSA readings, bone scans and visits. As ADT is associated with osteoporosis, bone den-sity studies will be required along with a regime to lessen bone loss, such as supplemental Vitamin D, calcium, bisphosphonates, or the more powerful Xgeva (denosumab).

If there is still some evidence of disease progression, patients become candidates for chemotherapy with Taxotere (docetaxzel) or Jevtana (cabazitaxel). These patients also become candidates for the newly developed drugs, such as Zytiga (abiraterone), Xtandi (enzalutimide), Xofigo (radium Ra 223 dichloride), or Provenge (sipuleucel-T).

How and when to use these new drugs is a matter of debate. The emerging management is based on five parameters: PSA doubling time, symptoms or pain requiring more than Tylenol, bone metastases as indicated by a bone scan, performance status (a score from 1-5 with a good score meaning 0-1 according to the ECOG performance status (Eastern Cooperative Oncology Group), and history of prior use of chemotherapy. This permits categorization of patients into six categories. Let me define the six categories and what is recommended for each group.

CATEGORY 1

These patients will have rising PSA, no symptoms, no metastases, good performance status, and no prior chemotherapy. Such patients will be advised to be monitored, nothing more. If they are uncomfortable with this advice, they can be offered different anti-androgens, such as Casodex, Euflex, or Anandron. They can also be offered Nizoral (ketoconazole) with prednisone, a regime that inhibits androgen from being made by the adrenal gland.

CATEGORY 2

These patients will have rising PSA, have minimal or no symptoms, known metastases, good performance status, and no prior chemotherapy. These patients will be offered Zytiga (abiraterone 250 mg tablets 4 times a day along with prednisone 5 mg twice a day), or chemotherapy with Taxotere (docetaxel 75 mg/square M, IV every 3 weeks), or Provenge (sipuleucel-T), the $100,000 immunotherapy based on acid phosphatise, a protein specific to prostate cancer.

CATEGORY 3

These patients will have rising PSA, be symptomatic, have metastases, have good performance status, and no prior chemotherapy. These patients are candidates for Zytiga, or chemotherapy with docetaxel or Jevtana (cabazitaxel 25 mg/square M, IV every 3 weeks).

CATEGORY 4

These patients will have rising PSA, be symptomatic, have metastases, have poor performance status, and no prior chemotherapy. These patients are candidates for Zytiga and Xofigo (radium Ra 223 dichloride).

CATEGORY 5

These patients will have rising PSA, be symptomatic, have metastases, good performance status, and prior chemotherapy with doctaxel. These patients are candidates for Zytiga, Jevtana, or Xtandi.

CATEGORY 6

These patients will have rising PSA, be symptomatic, have metastases, poor performance status and prior chemotherapy. These patients are candidates for palliative care only.

In all categories, patients with known bone metastases will be prescribed calcium (1000 mg), vitamin D (800 IU) and Xgeva (denosumab 120 mg subcutaneously every 4 weeks).

This is what is done today. What the future holds is one big question mark. Will focal therapy, applying heat, like HIFU (High

Intensity Focused Ultrasound), or cold (creating ice balls) to affected portions of the prostate gland ever replace total removal of the prostate with or without robotic aid? Will low-grade electrical energy totally eradicate cancer? Will earlier use of drugs, like Zytiga or Xtandi, make surgery unnecessary? Will there ever be a vaccine to prevent the disease from occurring? How long will it take to answer some of these questions? Will there be an approach about which we can only dream today?

There is no doubt that this is a disease which will focus and direct our attention in the coming years. Prostate cancer remains a force which challenges our abilities to move from the treatment to the cure. As a surgeon, I have seen a gamut of emotions on the faces of my patients; from the fear which accompanies the initial diagnosis to the joy and relief which is the response to a zero PSA after surgery.

I have made it my life's work to strive for the latter in every one of my cases. Perhaps my only regret is that we are not given a lifespan of two hundred years. It would be wonderful to be there when the cure will be a certainty – in all cases!

Afterword

As an afterthought, I am going to wax philosophical and express candidly what I think about our health care system in Canada: what I think is good, what I think is bad, and how we might make the system work better.

First, some background.

I graduated from McGill medical school in 1959 and decided to become a urologist in 1960, which is more than a half a century ago. I qualified to practise the specialty in 1964 and started my practice in 1966. I am still at it, forty-eight years later, enjoying every moment of my working day. My entire career has been spent as an academic clinician at the adult teaching hospitals of McGill University – the Royal Victoria and the Montreal General hospital. I have been richly rewarded for my efforts being named "best teacher" by resident doctors one year, "best doctor" by colleagues in another and, although I neither sought it nor solicited it, there is a Taguchi Chair in Urology at McGill University endowed by a grateful and generous patient – Mr. Lucien Remillard. I can think of no greater honour.

What intrigued my interest in the field, first of all, was kidney failure and the emerging treatments of the day, these being dialysis and transplantation. I assisted in the very first haemodialysis done at the Royal Victoria Hospital and became involved in the cadaver source kidney transplantation program, the first in the country, launched at the Royal Vic. In the early days of haemodialysis, we had to reinforce all the connections to the tubing, which formed a significant part of the artificial kidney, and keep our eyes glued to the coils in the tub, Kelly forceps in hand, ready to clamp the in-flow and outflow, should there be a burst in the coil. I did that with my senior resident, Dr. Steve Helle, who has since had a long and distinguished career as a respected nephrologist.

Faced with the challenges of dialysis, I proposed exploring the lining of the small intestine as a dialyzing membrane in a procedure that was called the Taguchi loop. The idea was to substitute the sheet of cellophane, the essential element of the artificial kidney, with bowel lining, and bring "washing" fluid to it so that the waste or urine normally eliminated by the kidney would be washed out with the irrigating fluid pumped through it.

I gained notoriety as the procedure was tried in a number of hospitals in Canada. It had only limited success, though, because the inner lining of the small intestine, called intestinal villi, failed to remove sufficient amounts of uric acid and creatinine, two of the waste products that accumulate in the blood when the kidneys fail. The procedure did lower the need for regular connections to the artificial kidney, and it did correct water intoxication, acid balance, salt irregularities, and urea accumulation. This experiment was carried out before the development of the drug allopurinol, which lowers blood levels of uric acid in favour of its predecessor, xanthine, which dissolves more readily. The bowel dialysis might have worked better had allopurinol been available.

A word about the invention of the artificial kidney. Wilhelm Kolff was a young doctor in the Netherlands in the early 1940s when a young woman with severe kidney failure came under his care. He applied the treatment of the day, a magnesium sulphate enema in a darkened room. This lowered the blood pressure and reduced the chances of convulsions. There was nothing more to offer as the staff waited for the patient to fall into a coma and die.

Just at this time, Kolff attended a public lecture on semi-permeable membranes delivered by a physiologist, a certain Dr. Brinkman. Kolff heard the professor say that if solutions of different compositions were separated by a semi-permeable membrane, like cellophane, the composition will soon equalize, while larger molecules and products like blood cells would not pass through the "pores." In that juxtaposition of patient and lecture, the idea of the artificial kidney was born.

"What if I were to place the blood of my uremic patient inside a cellophane bag and place the bag inside a washtub filled with a solution that simulated normal serum?" Kolff wondered. He tried the experiment with his patient's blood, and it worked – the uremic serum became more normal. The cellophane tubing in Kolff's original artificial kidney was sausage casing obtained from a local butcher shop.

Subsequently, a search was launched for the equivalent of cellophane, or dialyzing membrane, within the human body. Small bowel lining was a contender, and one centre isolated a part of this structure to use just for dialysis. The small intestine was shortened by half its length, and the two ends of the isolated half were brought out to the skin. A solution that simulated serum was pumped in one opening, and the altered fluid was collected at the other end. This procedure worked, in principle, but only for a very short time. The small intestine appeared to require the transit of food and digestive enzymes in order to retain its fine capillary network.

What was new in my proposal was that I proposed to use the entire length of the small bowel by constructing Roux-Y joints at both the upper and lower ends. In a Roux-Y joint, the bowel is interrupted, the distal cut end is brought out to the skin, and the proximal cut end rejoined to the bowel a short distance further down. When this is done at the upper and lower end of the small intestine, the upper opening can be used to drip in dialyzing fluid, and a catheter inserted at the lower opening can be used to suck out the altered fluid. When the intestine is not used to substitute for the kidney, it should process food as it normally would and not regurgitate out the opening because of the one-way flow of the intestinal content, known as peristalsis. And, as I have indicated, we did have some success with the procedure.

Subsequently, I was assigned to help solve the transplant rejection problem. My solution was based on overwhelming the recipient animal with donor specific protein, and although I earned a PhD solving the problem of graft rejection in a rat kidney transplantation model, the experiment failed to work in dogs and thus, presumably, in man. Nevertheless, a technique I developed to connect the ureter to the bladder in the rat, which I tried out on a human recipient, was eminently successful. The technique was adopted by transplant centres in many other countries after urologists in Argentina determined that it was simpler to carry out and superior to other established methods. It is known today as the Taguchi U-stitch.

During my half-century exposure to urology, I have witnessed innumerable advances. Endoscopic surgery, with a camera that displays on a television screen what used to be seen by just one eye against the lens, has made the TURP (trans-urethral prostatic resection) and bladder tumour resection easier to carry out as well as to teach. The use of laser energy has made stone problems, bladder tumours, and even very large prostatic enlargements less burdensome for patients. Blocked kidneys and blocked ureters are routinely unblocked without skin-cutting operations. Surgical interventions, meanwhile, are expected to cure early cancers of the kidney, bladder, prostate, and testis.

Many procedures have disappeared from common practice. The Boyce procedure, wherein a kidney was literally bi-valved in order to extract a large stone, called a staghorn calculus, is seldom, if ever, done today. Partial removal of a kidney and even complete removal of a kidney harboring a cancerous mass has become a laparoscopic procedure; the skin-cutting operation reserved for those cases where the cancer has spread to the main body vein called the vena cava.

Skin-cutting procedures to remove stones from the ureter have been abandoned, as have bikini cuts to correct stress-incontinence in women. Urologists remain the surgeons of the urinary tracts of women and of the urinary and genital tracts of men. In large academic centres, each urologist has become a sub-specialist: an example would be that of a urologic oncologist, or one who devotes all his time to andrology, infertility, transplantation, incontinence, or stone disease.

I had the privilege of handling all urologic problems when I began my career but, in recent years, settled on prostate disorders when it became necessary to narrow the scope of practice.

It should be apparent from the above account that I have had a long and interesting career. But does success with clinical practice entitle one to comment on overall health care delivery in the country? Perhaps! Maybe not! Please hear me out.

The government-run universal Canadian Medicare program was introduced in 1968. It eliminated all discussion of who would pay for what, even when one catastrophic problem followed another. The insurance payment does not run out, as can be the problem with private insurance, no matter how good the plan, as is the case in the U.S. There can be abuse and dishonest claims certainly, but on the whole, the plan has worked exceedingly well. Canadians cannot understand why such a reassuring system is not in effect around the world. They cannot fathom why so many people in the U.S. oppose it.

Hospital use has changed, though. Hospitalization for frivolous disorders does not occur. Hospital stays for major operations have become dramatically shortened. Routinely, an open radical prostatectomy, for example, is a two-day hospitalization, TURP a one-day stay.

And yet, there are bed-shortages necessitating last minute cancellations of cases. How can that be?

The answer, in my view, lies in our failure to adapt to the revolutionary advances that have occurred. We live in a world where dialysis and even organ transplantation have no age limits, where life-saving medications cost hundreds of thousands of dollars per case, where disposable materials used in surgery often exceed the surgeon's fee.

But the way health care workers are rewarded in Canada has not changed. Doctors are still doing piecework: the more they do, the more they get, the less they do, the less they earn. Nurses are on fixed salaries, the pay scale related to years of experience more than to any other criterion. And administrators are government employees rewarded more for coming in on budget than for the quality and quantity of services provided.

How can a system work where the three main players, doctors, nurses and administrators, are not working hand-in-hand? To be frank, they are not even on the same page!

What do I mean by that?

Let's get back to the case cancelled because there were "no beds." "No beds" does not refer to actual beds. There are plenty of beds not in use. "No beds" is a euphemism for "no nurses." And "no nurses" is in evidence because the administration fails to hire the necessary number. It does so to cut services, in order to come in on budget. Employing more nurses and doing more procedures escalates costs and endangers the carefully prepared budget. The administration is simply fulfilling its mandate.

Meanwhile, the cancelled patient is not at all pleased. He has prepared for the date, probably cleaned out his bowel with an enema, possibly invited out-of-town relatives to be in town. He is certain that if he were a VIP, a CEO of a major firm, he would not be cancelled. And, of course, he is right! The surgeon is also upset. The last-minute cancellation means he cannot schedule office visits in its place. He cannot generate income. Nor can the anaesthesiologist. The operating room lies dormant, including all the staff that normally staff the theatre.

That is what I mean when I say administration, nurses, and surgeons are not working together – not on the same page.

What is the solution? In a utopian world, socialism might be the answer. In such a society, people would be rewarded equally, regardless of effort or complexity of challenges. But that is not the world in which we live.

Ours is a free but competitive society in which acceptance into medical school is highly prized, residency-training programs compete for the best graduates, and institutions strive to outdo the competition. Our society is built on healthy competition, but we have abandoned competition in running our hospitals. We have concentrated instead on building modern 1000-plus bed monster hospitals, when the data have shown that large hospitals are inefficient. Studies in the U.S. reveal that 500-bed hospitals work best.

We should be building 500-bed hospitals that compete with one another for best services, best results. To achieve this, doctors, nurses, and administrators must work together, not independently of one another, as is the case today, and the government must reward those institutions which prove to be superior. Simple logic, it seems to me.

Best services, best results may not be so easy to measure, to be sure. Teaching hospitals wherein students and residents learn their trade cannot operate as efficiently as institutions where trainees do not "get in the way." Nor are all cases of the same disease the same. A more complex or complicated case cannot be expected to have the same course as one that is more straightforward. Still, an audit can determine that. Volume of work, outcomes, complication rates, patient satisfaction, costs per case, and staff satisfaction are all measurable parameters. Institutions that perform well must reward every category of worker, not just the professionals. There should be an incentive to outdo the competition, and this work ethic must be pervasive throughout the entire institution.

It can be argued that modern medicine's need for expensive equipment, like the Da Vinci robot, PET scanner, MRI, shock-wave stone crusher, etc., cannot be installed in every 500-bed hospital. Agreed, but expensive technology can be distributed reasonably and fairly.

Is healthy competition for best services a pipe dream? Perhaps, but not at all impossible to implement in my estimation! Nor am I alone in proposing healthy competition as a way to improve health care. In their 2006 book, *Redefining Health Care* (Harvard Business Review Press), Michael E. Porter and Elizabeth Olmstead Teisberg examined health care in the U.S. and found much at fault. "Health care is on a collision course between patient needs and economic reality," they claimed. "Value-based competition on results" is the only logical solution, they conclude.

If that has any hope of succeeding in the U.S., it should be ten times easier to implement in Canada.